9/87

CANCER IN ATOMIC BOMB SURVIVORS

GANN Monograph on Cancer Research

The "GANN Monograph on Cancer Research" series is promoted by the Japanese Cancer Association. This semiannual series of monographs was initiated in 1966 by the late Dr. Tomizo Yoshida (1903–1973) and is now published jointly by Japan Scientific Societies Press, Tokyo and Plenum Press, New York and London. Each volume consists of collected contributions on current topics in cancer problems and allied research fields. The publication of these monographs owes much to the financial support given by the late Professor Kazushige Higuchi, the Jikei University School of Medicine.

The planning for each volume is done by the Board of Executive Directors of the Japanese Cancer Association, with the final approval of the Board of Directors. It is hoped that the series will serve as an important source of information in the field of cancer research.

Japanese Cancer Association

JAPANESE CANCER ASSOCIATION

GANN Monograph on Cancer Research No.32

CANCER IN ATOMIC BOMB SURVIVORS

Edited by

ITSUZO SHIGEMATSU
Radiation Effects Research Foundation, Hiroshima, Japan
ABRAHAM KAGAN
Radiation Effects Research Foundation, Hiroshima, Japan

JAPAN SCIENTIFIC SOCIETIES PRESS, Tokyo
PLENUM PRESS, New York and London

August 1986

Published jointly by
JAPAN SCIENTIFIC SOCIETIES PRESS
2-10 Hongo, 6-chome, Bunkyo-ku, Tokyo 113, Japan
ISBN 4-7622-9490-X
          and
PLENUM PRESS
233 Spring Street, New York, NY 10013, USA
ISBN 0-306-42501-7

Distributed in all areas outside Japan and Asia between Pakistan and Korea by PLENUM PRESS, New York and London.

Printed in Japan

PREFACE

Follow-up studies of persons exposed to medical radiation have long shown that radiation induces cancer in man. This, coupled with increasing exposure from other sources including occupational and environmental radiations, has resulted in greater recognition of the importance of research on radiation-induced carcinogenesis and risk assessment with a view to radiation protection.

One of the well-known late effects of radiation is the increased incidence of leukemia that occurred among atomic bomb survivors beginning two or three years after exposure. A remarkable increase of solid tumors including cancers of the thyroid, breast and lung was also observed 10 to 20 years after exposure. Thus, many pathological, clinical and epidemiological studies have been made on radiation carcinogenesis in atomic bomb survivors by investigators at the Atomic Bomb Casualty Commission (ABCC), now known as the Radiation Effects Research Foundation (RERF), as well as by the staff of universities in Hiroshima and Nagasaki. Some of the mechanisms involved in radiation carcinogenesis in man and associated modifying factors, such as age at time of exposure and sex, have been elucidated by these studies. The results obtained are being used by such agencies as the International Commission on Radiation Protection (ICRP) for risk estimations of radiation exposure.

This monograph presents the results realized thus far in these epidemiological and pathological studies. The incidence of radiation-induced cancer among atomic bomb survivors continues to be high 40 years after exposure, and much remains unknown about radiation carcinogenesis. It is hoped that this publication will stimulate the promotion of further studies.

Questions were raised recently on the dosimetry system which has been used as the basis for estimating the risks of carcinogenesis in atomic bomb survivors. As a consequence, a joint reassessment was undertaken some years ago by the U. S. and Japan.

It had been hoped that this radiation dosimetry reassessment, the status of which was reported and discussed at workshops in 1981, 1983 and 1985, would be available for the analyses presented in this monograph. Regrettably, due to the complex nature of the matter a report at the workshop in March 1986 stated that completion of the task was still several months away. Further delay, therefore, in release of this monograph does not appear justified.

It is clear from earlier reports that the estimated radiation dose from neutrons will be sharply reduced and that the estimated gamma dose will increase in Hiroshima, but will decrease slightly in Nagasaki. The shape of the dose-response curve and magnitude of risk coefficients may be altered slightly, but preliminary analyses based on incomplete data suggest that no major change will occur in the determination of the relation of radiation to cancer occurrence.

Many people have contributed to the production of this monograph. In particular, vi

we wish to commend Dr. Hiroo Kato, Dr. Suminori Akiba, and Mr. Geoffrey Day for their invaluable editorial assistance and Mrs. Merry Y. Uemoto for her expert word processing.

May 1986

I. SHIGEMATSU
A. KAGAN

CONTENTS

SAMPLING OF ATOMIC BOMB SURVIVORS AND METHOD OF CANCER DETECTION IN HIROSHIMA AND NAGASAKI

Itsuzo Shigematsu and Suminori Akiba

*Radiation Effects Research Foundation**

The number of acute deaths in both cities which occurred due to the atomic bombings of Hiroshima and Nagasaki in August 1945 until the end of December 1945 is estimated to be between 150,000–200,000 and the number of survivors identified by the supplementary schedule of the 1950 National Census is 284,000. From among these survivors, a fixed population, the Life Span Study (LSS) sample, was established and has been followed by the Atomic Bomb Casualty Commission-the Radiation Effects Research Foundation (ABCC-RERF). In this paper the sampling methods of the fixed population are explained. Also described is the utilization of the tumor and tissue registries in Hiroshima and Nagasaki, the LSS and the Adult Health Study (AHS) for cancer detection among the fixed population.

Atomic bombs (A-bombs) were dropped on Hiroshima and Nagasaki in August 1945. The damage in the two cities was caused by a combination of heat, blast, and fire. The total area demolished by these causes was about 13 km² in Hiroshima and 7 km² in Nagasaki. The energy of the Nagasaki bomb exceeded that of the Hiroshima bomb, but the burned-out areas of Hiroshima were greater because of differences of topography and of the distribution of buildings (Fig. 1).

The number of A-bomb related acute deaths which occurred before the end of December 1945 is estimated to be somewhere between 90,000 and 120,000 out of a population of approximately 330,000 in Hiroshima and between 60,000 and 80,000 out of about 250,000 in Nagasaki (Fig. 1). These acute deaths were attributable to A-bomb radiation, burns, and/or mechanical injuries.

The Atomic Bomb Casualty Commission (ABCC) was established in the two cities by the United States government in 1947 to initiate follow-up studies on the late health effects of A-bomb radiation. ABCC was soon joined in its studies by a branch laboratory of the Japanese National Institute of Health.

In 1975, responsibility for these studies was assumed by the Radiation Effects Research Foundation (RERF), an independent binational institution equally funded by the governments of Japan and the United States.

A nationwide survey of A-bomb survivors was first conducted in 1950, identifying a total of 284,000 survivors throughout the country. A sample of about 110,000 subjects was selected from among these survivors and nonexposed controls who were resident in Hiroshima and Nagasaki at the time of the survey.

As indicated in Table I, mortality in this Life Span Study (LSS) sample has been

---

* Hijiyama Park 5-2, Minami-ku, Hiroshima 732, Japan (重松逸造, 秋葉澄伯).

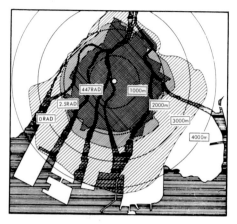 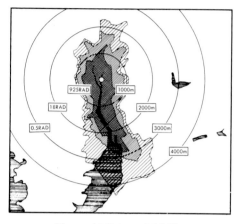

Hiroshima 6 August 1945   Nagasaki 9 August 1945

Uranium-235 15 kiloton TNT   Plutonium-239 21 kiloton TNT
Estimated population 330,000   Estimated population 250,000
Acute deaths during 1945 90,000-120,000   Acute deaths during 1945 60,000-80,000

FIG. 1.   A-bomb damage in Hiroshima and Nagasaki. ○, ground zero; ▓, extent of fire; ▒, mean line of structural damage; ▨, limit of structural damage.

under study since 1958, and autopsies (Pathology Study) have also been performed on many of the individuals who have died. Since 1958, detailed biennial medical examinations have been carried out at a participation rate of 75%–85% on an LSS subsample, the Adult Health Study (AHS) sample, comprising about 20,000 members. A separate sample of 2,800 children exposed in utero and their nonexposed controls has been followed for mortality and morbidity.

TABLE I.   Major ABCC-RERF Programs

Program	Number of subjects	Year base population obtained	Year study initiated
Survivors			
Life Span	110,000	1950	1958
Pathology	70,000	1950	1962
Adult Health	20,000	1950	1958
In utero	2,800	1945–46	1956
Offspring			
F_1 mortality	77,000	1946–	1960
Biochemical genetics	45,000	1946–	1975
Cytogenetics	33,000	1946–	1967

Program	Type of study	Year study initiated
Other studies		
Immunology	Tumor markers and immune response	1980
Experimental pathology	Cell biology	1979
Cerebrovascular diseases (CVD) (Ni-Hon-San)	Japanese in Hiroshima-Nagasaki, Honolulu, and San Francisco	1969
Cancer	Breast, Lung, Colorectal	1979
Reassessment of A-bomb dosimetry	Japan-US joint study	1981

A large scale genetic study was also conducted based on pregnancy registrations in both Hiroshima and Nagasaki during 1948–53. Furthermore, a sample consisting of 77,000 children whose parents were either exposed or nonexposed was set up in 1960 for mortality follow-up and later for cytogenetic and biochemical genetic studies.

Besides these studies, other programs such as immunological studies and the reassessment of A-bomb dosimetry have been developed (Table I).

Sampling of A-bomb Survivors for Follow-up Study

The earliest, reliable, large sample of A-bomb survivors was defined by the supplementary schedules of the 1950 National Census, totaling about 284,000 survivors, of whom about 159,000 were in Hiroshima and about 125,000 in Nagasaki at the time of the bombs (ATB). Only subjects who were residents of Hiroshima (98,000) and Nagasaki (97,000) in 1950 were used in constructing the Master Sample from which the LSS and AHS subsamples were drawn (3). The composition of the Master Sample is shown in Table II. Briefly, the Master Sample consists of two parts; the proper part and the reserve part. The reserve part has the same characteristics as the proper part such as Japanese citizen and known Koseki (family register), but differs in that the Honseki (place of permanent family registration) is outside their immediate environs of Hiroshima or Nagasaki Cities. The proper part was further classified into two parts: "selected" for the LSS sample and "not selected" which was not selected by random sampling in the matching process by exposure distance.

All cases in the Master Sample proper part who were within 2,500 m from ground zero ATB were selected for the LSS sample, with the 28,130 subjects within 2,000 m from ground zero serving as the core of the sample. An equal number of subjects who were between 2,500–9,999 m from ground zero and those not in the cities (NIC) ATB were selected to match the core group by sex and age. However, as the NIC subjects

TABLE II. Proper and Reserve Parts of the Master Sample by Component, Exposure Category, and City

City	Exposure category		Total	Proper part		Reserve part
				Selected	Not selected	
Hiroshima		Total	121,100	74,356	16,341	30,403
	A	0–1,999 m from ground zero	26,174	21,329	—	4,845
	B	2,000–2,499 m	14,543	11,524	—	3,019
	C[a]	2,500–9,999 m	44,478	21,275	14,748	8,455
	D[a]	10,000+ m or Not in City	35,905	20,228	1,593	14,084
Nagasaki		Total	42,620	25,037	10,458	7,125
	A	0–1,999 m from ground zero	7,659	6,801	—	858
	B	2,000–2,499 m	5,949	5,144	—	805
	C[a]	2,500–9,999 m	18,152	6,742	8,900	2,510
	D[a]	10,000+ m or Not in City	10,860	6,350	1,558	2,952
Total		Total	163,720	99,393	26,799	37,528
	A	0–1,999 m from ground zero	33,833	28,130	—	5,703
	B	2,000–2,499 m	20,492	16,668	—	3,824
	C[a]	2,500–9,999 m	62,630	28,017	23,648	10,965
	D[a]	10,000+ m or Not in City	46,765	26,578	3,151	17,036

[a] Matched by age and sex to Group A.

TABLE III. Number of Subjects in the Extended LSS Sample

Exposure		Hiroshima	Nagasaki	Total
Total		82,081	26,679	108,760
Nonexposed (Not in City)		20,170	6,348	26,518
Exposed	0 rad	27,577	4,004	31,581
	1–9	15,933	7,140	23,073
	10–99	13,694	5,473	19,167
	100–199	1,740	1,388	3,128
	200+	1,538	1,369	2,907
	Unknown	1,429	957	2,386

were not available from the 1950 National Census, they were selected from the 1st and 2nd ABCC 10% Sample Censuses in 1950–51 and the 1953 Daytime Census for Hiroshima, the 1950 Listing of Family Heads, the 1950 City Consumer's Registry, and the ABCC 10% Sample Census in 1950 for Nagasaki. Thus, a total of 99,393 subjects constitute the initial LSS sample (Table II). Later, in 1970, all the reserve part of the Master Sample within 2,500 m from ground zero (9,367 persons) were added to the LSS sample in order to enlarge the proximally exposed groups (6). Thus, the Extended LSS sample consists of 108,760 subjects as shown in Table III by dose and city.

Another source of information about A-bomb survivors is the A-bomb handbook for which detailed explanation is given elsewhere (1). The purpose of issuing the handbook is to identify the A-bomb survivors based on the Atomic Bomb Survivors Medical Treatment Law which was enacted in 1957 for administrative purposes. Information on A-bomb radiation exposure status for the A-bomb handbook is based on the report made by the subject at the time of handbook issue, i.e., 1957 or later. Initially, medical care was limited by the law to the proximally exposed. Later, many persons who entered the cities immediately after the bombing, the so-called early entrants, were also included as A-bomb handbook holders. Thus, the total number of A-bomb handbook holders was about 370,000 as of March 1984 (1). It is believed that the exposure information from the A-bomb handbook is less accurate and not as complete as that ascertained for the ABCC-RERF sample. Also, estimation by the most reliable method of exposure dose from A-bomb radiation is virtually limited to survivors belonging to the RERF sample. Thus, the results of surveys referred to in this monograph are limited to those conducted on the ABCC-RERF samples unless otherwise specified.

Method of Cancer Detection

1. Tumor and tissue registry

A) Tumor registry

Tumor Registries were established in 1957 for Hiroshima and in 1958 for Nagasaki under the auspices of the respective City Medical Associations and with the technical support of ABCC (5). The specific purpose was to develop and maintain a source of information on tumors diagnosed in these two communities. They have been, and continue to be, effective mechanisms for the collection and storage of cancer case information, and the data recorded have been invaluable in the assessment of the role of ionizing radiation in the etiology of certain specific cancers, particularly nonfatal cancer.

B) *Tissue registry*

The Tissue Registries are designed to collect and examine surgical tumor tissue from both Hiroshima and Nagasaki subjects. Tumors are classified and the tissues are stored. This procedure permits reexamination of tissues by investigators for specific research projects. The Tissue Registry was established in Hiroshima in 1973 under the auspices of the Hiroshima Prefectural Medical Association (thus the Tissue Registry covers tumor tissue removed during surgery conducted in Hiroshima prefecture including Hiroshima City). A similar Tissue Registry was initiated by the Nagasaki City Medical Association in September 1974.

The information for tumor cases registered in the Tumor and/or Tissue Registry who are LSS members becomes available by checking the names in the registry against the RERF Master File once a year.

The completeness of registration appears to be high, judging from the low proportion of cases which were registered only upon death certificate information (9% in Hiroshima and 7% in Nagasaki). However, overregistration may occur because of the inclusion of doubtful diagnoses, and occult cancer. In order to reduce the false negative rate in screening cases for the cancer registry, a diagnosis described as doubtful by the attending physician is so registered, unless it is corrected or confirmed by a later report. As mentioned earlier, the autopsy rate is high in Hiroshima and Nagasaki, particularly in the RERF sample, so therefore the number of occult cancer (recognized only at autopsy) is also high. The consequence of such overregistration will be described later in this monograph. The Tumor Registry data are limited to sample members who lived in Hiroshima and Nagasaki cities or adjacent areas at the time of diagnosis, whereas the

TABLE IV.   Accuracy of Cause of Death—Autopsy Cases among the LSS Sample, 1961–75

Cause of death	Death certifi-cate	Autopsy report	Agree-ment	Confir-mation rate (%)	Detec-tion rate (%)
Tuberculosis	176	226	110	62.5	48.7
Malignant neoplasms of:					
Buccal cavity and pharynx	19	17	13	68.4	76.5
Esophagus	50	53	36	72.0	67.9
Stomach	444	495	374	84.2	75.6
Large intestine	43	54	28	65.1	51.9
Rectum	45	46	32	71.1	69.6
Liver, gallbladder and bile ducts	42	169	26	61.9	15.4
Pancreas	56	81	36	64.3	44.4
Trachea, bronchus, lung	192	172	117	60.9	68.0
Breast	40	49	38	95.0	77.6
Uterus	70	83	57	81.4	68.7
Prostate	13	24	5	38.5	20.8
Urinary organs	38	60	30	78.9	50.0
Malignant lymphoma	40	56	31	77.5	55.4
Leukemia	42	40	36	85.7	90.0
Benign neoplasms and neoplasms of unspecified nature	65	21	3	4.6	14.3
Diseases of blood and blood-forming organs	30	14	12	40.0	85.7
Ischemic heart disease	265	199	67	25.3	33.7
Gastric, duodenal, and peptic ulcer	58	61	24	41.4	39.3
Cirrhosis of liver	153	149	80	52.3	53.7
Nephritis and nephrosis	62	29	11	17.7	37.9

mortality data cover subjects from all Japan. Since migration rates do not differ by radiation dose according to recent analyses of the AHS (8), this difference should not cause a serious problem in analysis of radiation induced cancer. However, a more detailed study of this problem of migration will be undertaken in the future.

2. The Life Span Study (LSS): a mortality survey

In Japan, all vital demographic events such as births, deaths, and marriages are registered at the legal address of the family (Honseki). This family registration system (Koseki) has been operating for more than 100 years. Therefore, it is possible to ascertain accurately the survival status of a person by checking the family register through the Honseki regardless of actual residence. Nearly all deaths in the LSS sample have been verified through the Koseki check and the cause of death is obtained from the vital statistics death schedules kept at the Health Center which covers the location at death. As the death certificate is used to prepare the death schedules, the accuracy of the cause classification must be checked against the autopsy report whenever possible. Table IV shows, in terms of confirmation and detection rates, the accuracy of the cause of death classification on death certificates as revealed by autopsy findings for those individuals who were autopsied (9). Confirmation rates differ according to the cause of death; the rate is high for cancer such as leukemia, lung, and stomach, being 70%–80%, but the accuracy is poor for cancer such as pancreas and liver where the confirmation rate is less than 50%. In studying cancer of sites having low accuracy, it is possible to restrict the study to only those histologically confirmed either through autopsy or surgical pathology.

The underlying cause of death is classified according to the International Classification of Diseases (ICD). The cause of death was coded by the 7th (1950–67), 8th (1968–78), and 9th (1979 or later) ICD revisions.

3. The Adult Health Study (AHS): a clinical survey

Regular biennial clinical examinations of the AHS sample which began in 1958 are now in the 14th examination cycle (1984). Sample selection and characteristics of the AHS are described elsewhere (2, 4). The original AHS population of almost 20,000 included two exposed and two control groups of approximately equal numbers as given in Table V: 1) a group within 2,000 m from ground zero, who reported acute radiation symptoms; 2) another group within 2,000 m, without acute radiation symptoms; 3) a control group between 3,000–3,499 m in Hiroshima and 3,000–3,999 m in Nagasaki; and 4) another control group not in the city ATB. Groups 2, 3, and 4 were matched to Group 1 by age and sex. The examination schedule was set so that in any one month a more or less representative cross section of the entire population would visit the clinic. Over time,

TABLE V.   The AHS Sample by Sex, City, and Exposure Group

Exposure group	Hiroshima		Nagasaki		Both cities		Total
	Male	Female	Male	Female	Male	Female	
1. Within 2,000 m with symptoms	1,312	2,116	678	887	1,990	3,003	4,993
2. Within 2,000 m without symptoms	1,313	2,114	677	883	1,990	2,997	4,987
3. 3,000–3,499 m in Hiroshima 3,000–3,999 m in Nagasaki	1,312	2,119	674	885	1,986	3,004	4,990
4. Not in city ATB	1,313	2,120	676	883	1,989	3,003	4,992
Total	5,250	8,469	2,705	3,538	7,955	12,007	19,962

attrition (death, moved from city, and refusal) has reduced the population examined in 1984 to about 50% of the original sample.

The medical examination in the clinic is a standard one, consisting of a system review, physical findings, and up to six diagnoses according to ICD nomenclature, all coded. Other basic clinical data at the time of the examination are systolic and diastolic blood pressure, height and weight, and electrocardiogram and chest film diagnoses, all coded. Ultrasonography of the abdomen, begun in Hiroshima in 1982, is performed regularly on about 50% of the AHS, while of these, 75% also have a thyroid examination, and about 60% (females) a breast examination.

In addition to routine laboratory tests, specific biochemical and immunological assay for cancer screening was recorded. Included among these procedures are serum pepsinogen and anti parietal antibody for stomach cancer and α-fetoprotein and HB-s antigen for liver cancer.

The clinical diagnoses available for the AHS are difficult to characterize, especially if they are not based on laboratory findings. Most investigators have used the coded diagnoses for initial ascertainment only, reexamining the patient or reviewing the medical records to make final selections in relation to study criteria. There is little information on the frequency with which diagnoses are missed. The ascertainment varies also in relation to the special interests and experience of the examiners, the existence of particular substudies, and other factors.

On Limitations of Data

Although these epidemiological studies included control groups for comparative purposes, it was not possible to set up an ideal population sample (7). For example, the number of survivors exposed near ground zero is limited, and cannot be augmented. The selection of a proper control group presents another problem. Essentially, any control group should resemble the experimental group in every respect except the factors being tested (radiation exposure in this case). Because everyone in the area was exposed to some degree and subject to blast effects and burns, a sample was taken of the population residing in the city at the time of the survey who were not in the cities ATB. The NIC group was subdivided into early and late entrants into the cities since they might have represented different kinds of populations. Actually, the NIC group appears to differ from the A-bomb survivors in other respects such as socioeconomic status. Therefore, in many instances, the NIC group has been abandoned as a control in favor of survivors with very low exposure doses, for example, 0, or 0–9 rad.

The studies involving the major samples are based on the A-bomb survivors who were still alive at the initial survey about five years after the bombs. Therefore, the samples exclude the more severely injured, and offer the possibility of measuring the delayed effects of exposure, from light to moderately heavy radiation doses.

Sample size poses a problem. When the data are classified by city, sex, age, radiation exposure, and cause of illness or cause of death, the frequency of events dwindles very rapidly. This introduces variability into the data, and creates difficulties in their interpretation. Inferences can be made only after the performance of statistical tests of significance to give some assurance that the differences observed are not due to chance alone.

REFERENCES

1. A-bomb Casualty Relief Department, Public Health Bureau, Hiroshima City. "Gembaku Hibakusha Taisaku Jigyo Gaiyo, Showa 59 Nen-ban (General Description of Projects to Help A-bomb Survivors, Annual Report 1984)."

2. Beebe, G.W., Fujisawa, H., and Yamasaki, M. Adult Health Study. Reference papers. A. Selection of the sample. B. Characteristics of the sample. ABCC Tech. Rep. 10-60 (1960).

3. Beebe, G. W. and Usagawa, M. The major ABCC samples. ABCC Tech. Rep. 12-68 (1968).

4. Hollingsworth, J. W. and Beebe, G. W. Adult Health Study, provisional research plan. ABCC Tech. Rep. 9-60 (1960).

5. Ishida, M., Zeldis, L. J., and Jablon, S. Tumor registry study in Hiroshima and Nagasaki. ABCC Tech. Rep. 2-61 (1961).

6. Kato, H. and Schull, W. Life Span Study Report 9. Part 1. Cancer mortality among atomic bomb survivors, 1950–78. RERF Tech. Rep. 12-80 (1980).

7. Moriyama, I. M. Capsule summary of results of radiation studies on Hiroshima and Nagasaki atomic bomb survivors, 1945–75. RERF Tech. Rep. 5-77 (1977).

8. Sawada, H., Kodama, K., Shimizu, Y., and Kato, H. RERF Adult Health Study, Report 6. Result of the six examination cycles, 1968–80, Hiroshima and Nagasaki. RERF Tech. Rep. 3-86 (1986).

9. Yamamoto, T., Moriyama, I. M., Asano, M. and Guralnick, L. RERF Pathology Studies, Report 4. Autopsy program and the Life Span Study, Hiroshima and Nagasaki, January 1961–December 1975. RERF Tech. Rep. 18-78 (1978).

ATOMIC BOMB DOSIMETRY FOR EPIDEMIOLOGICAL STUDIES OF SURVIVORS IN HIROSHIMA AND NAGASAKI

Takashi Maruyama*

Division of Physics, National Institute of Radiological Sciences

Better atomic bomb (A-bomb) radiation dose estimates with a higher accuracy are required for the epidemiological studies in Hiroshima and Nagasaki. Several scientists have tried to evaluate the free-in-air gamma ray and neutron dose and some weighting factors such as house shielding and body shielding. Since 1965, the tentative 1965 dose (T65D) has been widely used as the basic data for the dose determination of A-bomb survivors in epidemiological studies.

In 1976, however, the reevaluation of the T65D dose was proposed by an American scientist who calculated the A-bomb doses on the basis of declassified data on the radiation spectra of the A-bomb. The development of computer technology made it possible to perform complicated dose-calculations for the Hiroshima and Nagasaki bombs.

This paper describes the history of A-bomb dosimetry, reviews some issues in the determination of T65D, and discusses the necessity of reassessment of A-bomb dose and the expected values for survivors.

By 1955 the Atomic Bomb Casualty Commission (ABCC) had accumulated a large body of medical information on the survivors in Hiroshima and Nagasaki. Most survivors were exposed to the atomic bombs (A-bombs) inside Japanese houses. According to ABCC investigations, Japanese houses were highly uniform in construction such as slope, thickness, and composition of the roofs, thickness and composition of the interior and exterior walls, and type and arrangement of framing. To determine the shielding factors typical Japanese houses were built at the Nevada Test Site and used during dosimetry studies in the Ichiban Project (3).

The early dose estimates for each survivor were determined on the basis of the tentative 1957 dose (T57D), the so-called York curves, which made the evaluations using results of A-bomb experiments at the Nevada Test Site (28). Since there were large errors in the dose determination because of uncertainties in the yield estimates of the bombs, the location of the explosion points, and various parameters in evaluating shielding, dose estimates with a higher degree of accuracy were desired. To revise the T57D, ABCC, in 1957, asked the Oak Ridge National Laboratory (ORNL) and the National Institute of Radiological Sciences (NIRS) for reevaluation of A-bomb doses. In 1965, ORNL and NIRS determined free-in-air doses for gamma rays and neutrons in Hiroshima and Nagasaki which were used to construct the tentative 1965 dose (T65D) (24). The current individual doses of A-bomb survivors in the ABCC/Radiation Effects

* Anakawa-cho 4-9-1, Chiba 260, Japan (丸山隆司).

Research Foundation (RERF) Life Span Study (LSS) sample have been evaluated on the basis of the T65D.

In 1976, Preeg of the Los Alamos National Laboratory (LANL) calculated free-in-air gamma ray and neutron doses, using the neutron and gamma ray output spectra of both the Hiroshima and Nagasaki bombs which were declassified by the US Energy Research and Development Administration and were published as a letter (36). Although the results of the dose calculations were not valid, they encouraged scientists to re-evaluate the A-bomb doses in Hiroshima and Nagasaki using the declassified output spectra. In 1980, Kerr (17, 18) of ORNL, and Loewe and Mendelsohn (20) of Lawrence Livermore National Laboratory (LLNL) calculated free-in-air gamma ray and neutron doses, using the output spectra proposed by Preeg. The ORNL and the LLNL reevaluations of the A-bombs in Hiroshima and Nagasaki were discussed at the Late Effects Workshop on Dosimetry of the Atomic Bomb Survivors (30) in 1981. Furthermore, a symposium entitled Reevaluations of Dosimetric Factors, Hiroshima and Nagasaki (34), was held under the auspices of the US Department of Energy in 1981 to evaluate past, present, and projected work on the A-bomb dosimetry. At these meetings it was impossible to determine which dose estimate is valid, the T65 dose or the revised dose by ORNL and LLNL. After these meetings, the US committee (Chairman: Dr. Seitz, Rockfeller University) and the Japanese committee (Chairman: Dr. Tajima, Rikkyo University) on reevaluation of the A-bomb doses were almost simultaneously established to decide an agreed best estimate of dose to survivors.

The first US-Japan Joint Workshop for Reassessment of Atomic Bomb Radiation Dosimetry in Hiroshima and Nagasaki was held in Nagasaki in February of 1983. At this workshop, new data on the gamma ray and neutron output spectra for the Hiroshima bomb evaluated with two-dimensional calculations were presented by Whalen (37). Kerr et al. (19) revised the gamma ray and neutron doses in Hiroshima which were previously published, with a dose recalculation on the basis of the new spectra calculated by Whalen. In November of 1983, the second US-Japan Joint Workshop was held in Hiroshima. At the second workshop a dosimetry system for A-bomb survivors including house shielding factors and organ dosimetric procedures was mainly discussed (27).

The Tentative 1965 Dose (T65D) Estimates

1. Characteristics of the A-bombs

The Nagasaki bomb was an implosion-type weapon that used thick charges of high explosive to compress a subcritical mass of ^{239}Pu into a critical mass at the time of explosion (Fig. 1). The implosion-type bomb was fired at Alamogordo in July 1945, at the Bikini Able test in 1946, and in several other tests at the Nevada Test Site. The Hiroshima bomb was a gun-assembly weapon that used a small propellant charge to shoot one piece of ^{235}U as a bullet against another piece to create a critical mass (Fig. 1). Since this type of bomb had never been fired at any other time, the dose estimates for Hiroshima were much more approximate as compared with those for Nagasaki. The mass and atomic number of materials surrounding the fissionable core are essential factors for the evaluation of radiation yield and quality. In the Nagasaki bomb, the surrounding materials contained high explosive of which hydrogen and nitrogen slowed down and absorbed most of the neutrons and consequently produced an intense source of high energy gamma rays. In the Hiroshima bomb, the iron and heavier metals used in parts

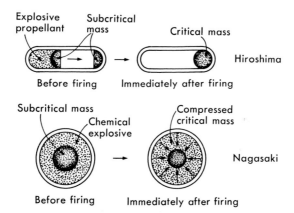

FIG. 1. Schematic illustration of construction of the Hiroshima and Nagasaki atomic bombs.

of the nose and tail of the bomb slowed down many fast neutrons and absorbed gamma rays, so that the neutron doses at corresponding distances from ground zero were thought to be very large as compared with those in Nagasaki. The radiation dose on the ground decreased rapidly with increasing distance from the burst point of the bomb due to geometrical and atmospheric attenuation.

2. *Exponential function for dose estimations*

According to the results of early A-bomb tests (*6*), gamma ray and neutron doses were given as a function of slant distance from the point of detonation at various distances above the air/ground interface by the following equation (Fig. 2):

$$D(R) = \frac{G_0 \exp\left(-R/L\right)}{R^2} \tag{1}$$

where $D(R)$ is free-in-air dose in rad at a slant distance R, L is the relaxation length in meters (m) for the type of radiations under consideration at a given air density, and G_0 is the intensity in rad·m² and is dependent on the particular type of A-bomb, yield, and type of radiation. During the early A-bomb tests, film badges and tetrachloro-ethylene chemical dosimeters were used to measure gamma ray doses, and neutron fluence distributions were determined with threshold detectors (*2*). It appeared likely that it would be difficult to determine precise radiation doses with these primitive detectors. Figure 3 shows the York curves, which were used for the dose determinations of

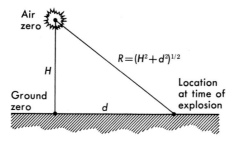

FIG. 2. Slant distance.

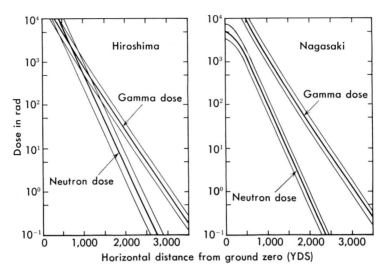

FIG. 3.   The York curves for the Hiroshima and Nagasaki bombs.

A-bomb survivors in Hiroshima and Nagasaki up to 1965. The methodology for the determinations of these curves is still unknown.

3. Operation BREN

To measure the gamma ray and neutron doses with sensitive laboratory-type instrumentation, the Bare Reactor Experiment, Nevada (BREN) was developed as a part of the Ichiban Project. The main objectives of Operation BREN were 1) to measure gamma ray and neutron doses in Japanese houses, 2) to determine the energy and angular distribution of gamma rays and neutrons, and 3) to measure energy and dose as functions of distance and height.

The Health Physics Research Reactor (HPRR) was designed to simulate the radiation field from an A-bomb. The HPRR was mounted on a 460 m-high tower constructed at the Nevada Test Site, and a ^{60}Co source of a nominal 1200 Ci (1 Ci$=$a 3.7×10^{10} Bq in SI unit) was substituted for the reactor to compensate gamma rays from fission products markedly attenuated in the reactor. As a part of the Ichiban Project, the LANL constructed a critical assembly designed to have nuclear characteristics similar to those of the Hiroshima bomb. Spectrum and dose measurements of neutrons from the critical assembly were carried out in the laboratory. The gamma ray dosimeter used during Operation BREN was the Phil, which is based on a miniature Geiger counter appropriately encapsulated so that its response per unit dose as a function of photon energy is uniform from an energy less than 100 keV to 10 MeV. The encapsulating shield included ^{6}Li to protect the detector from thermal neutrons to which it has a significant response (35). The neutron dosimeter used during Operation BREN was a Hurst proportional counter in conjunction with the appropriate electronics to provide a measure of approximate tissue kerma in air (14).

4. ORNL-Auxier

Since 1956, Auxier and his co-workers (Health Physics Division, ORNL) have conducted studies in conjunction with ABCC, aimed at determining the radiation dose

TABLE I. Dosimetric Parameters Used for the ORNL Dose Determinations (3)

Item	Hiroshima		Nagasaki	
	ORNL (1965)	York (1957)	ORNL (1965)	York (1957)
Energy yield, ktons of TNT equivalent	12.5	18.5	22	23
Height of burst (m)	570	550	500	519
Relaxation length (m)				
Neutrons	198	218	198	218
Gamma rays	250	346	350	346
Extrapolated G_0 at burst point (m² × rad)				
Neutrons	8.70×10^{10}	8.64×10^{10}	1.30×10^{10}	1.25×10^{10}
Gamma rays	3.45×10^{10}	2.16×10^{10}	2.75×10^{10}	2.68×10^{10}

York's and Wilson's values of G_0 have been converted to rad·cm² by multiplying by $(0.9144 \text{ m/yd})^2 \times$ (0.93 rad/R).

Relaxation length is corrected to 1.133 g/l., the surface air density in both cities at the time of the bombings.

Wilson gives only neutron fluxes. Values of G_0 for dose have been calculated from his fast fluxes assuming one-fast fission neutron per square centimeter delivers 1.14×10^{-9} rad.

Neutrons above 3 MeV and slow neutrons add only a few percent to the dose.

for survivors in Hiroshima and Nagasaki. They evaluated free-in-air doses of gamma rays and neutrons as a function of distances from ground zero, based on the results of Operation BREN and Ichiban experiments.

In Nagasaki, using the best gamma ray dose estimates from early A-bomb tests and computing a least squares solution, the values of G_0 and L given in Eq. (1) were determined. These values are given in Table I.

In Hiroshima, since no similar bomb had been test fired, the factors of G_0 and L were determined using the results of Operation BREN and the critical assembly experiment. Auxier (3) assumed that for gamma rays the relaxation length for neutrons was the same as in Nagasaki, but for gamma rays the relaxation length was much less in Hiroshima than in Nagasaki because of the difference in the construction of the bombs. At that time, they assumed that the energy yield of the Hiroshima bomb was 12.5 ktons of trinitrotoluen (TNT) equivalent and 22 ktons for the Nagasaki bomb. The results of the critical assembly experiment showed that total neutrons per fission was 0.76 and neutron dose per fission was 7.71×10^{-17} rad fission^{-1} at 9.46 m. They calculated the factor of G_0 for Hiroshima neutrons as 1.25×10^{10} rad m^{-2} at 1 m (12.5 ktons × 1.45 × 10^{23} fission kton^{-1} × 7.71×10^{-17} rad fission^{-1} × 9.46² m²). The buildup factor for neutrons was derived from the data measured in Operation BREN and was equal to 6.96. Table I gives the resultant values of these factors.

5. NIRS and Kyoto University

In 1961, Hashizume et al. (13) of NIRS started a project to evaluate free-in-air doses of gamma rays and neutrons in Hiroshima and Nagasaki at the request of ABCC. The NIRS group evaluated the gamma ray doses by thermoluminescent methods, using bricks and ornamental tiles from buildings which were still standing in Hiroshima and Nagasaki. In addition, they estimated the neutron doses from the activation of cobalt in iron reinforcing bars embedded at a depth of about 8 cm from the surface of ferroconcrete buildings in both cities.

TABLE II.   Specific Activities of ^{60}Co in Iron Bars and Resultant Neutron Dose (NIRS)

City	Coordinates of samples	Distance from ground zero (m)	Incident angle (°)	Activity[a] cpm/mg Co	Neutron dose (rad)
Hiroshima	27.61×23.47	260	66.60	2.09±0.170	7,864
	27.54×23.81	640	44.54	0.324±0.0204	1,188
	27.30×23.89	779	41.69	0.146±0.0013	541
	27.50×46.12	1,180	27.65	0.0124±0.0023	51
Nagasaki	51.29×46.02	590	42.55	0.140±0.0066	514
	50.42×46.49	1,030	31.79	0.0127±0.0010	52

[a] The figures indicate the measured values in the summer of 1963.

TABLE III.   Thermoluminescent Yield of Bricks and Tiles and Resultant Gamma Ray Dose (NIRS)

City	Coordinates of samples	Distance from ground zero (m)	Incident angle (°)	Luminescence L	Gamma ray dose (rad)
Hiroshima	27.37×23.53	140	79.46	21.4±1.4	10,118
	27.53×23.51	155	11.64	26.3±1.0	9,990
	27.36×23.43	170	73.44	20.4±1.1	8,578
	27.70×23.33	415	57.60	18.9±0.9	4,065
	27.84×23.45	605	45.41	24.0±1.2	1,582
	27.90×23.43	710	40.46	29.0±2.4	1,043
	27.43×23.45	965	34.76	38.8±2.3	338
Nagasaki	51.00×46.13	95	12.00	160.0±4.0	24,311
	51.23×46.29	520	46.75	213.0±6.0	6,435
	50.60×46.33	635	38.73	40.8±0.2	4,240
	50.39×46.22	860	31.69	11.8±1.1	1,639
	50.38×46.20	875	30.72	21.8±1.3	1,471
	51.23×45.68	970	27.65	12.0±1.0	937
	51.24×45.68	1,020	26.57	70.0±1.4	824

A) Neutrons

Cobalt is contained in iron as an impurity though in a very minute quantity. ^{59}Co is activated when irradiated by thermal neutrons and becomes ^{60}Co, which has a half-life of 5.27 years and emits beta rays with a maximum energy of 0.3 MeV. For the measurement of extremely weak activity of ^{60}Co, a coincidence type of beta ray spectrometer was used. In order to reduce the effect of self-absorption of beta rays on the activity measurement, the cobalt elements in iron samples were chemically separated and the Co fraction was deposited on a platinum planchet by electroplating.

Assuming that the spectrum of neutrons at distances greater than 500 m from ground zero was composed of a fast neutron component having a similar energy spectrum to that of the HPRR at ORNL, free-in-air neutron doses per unit specific activity of ^{60}Co were determined with an experiment in which iron rods imbedded in the concrete blocks at nearly 8 cm deep from the surface were irradiated with neutrons from the HPRR at ORNL. Table II gives the resultant specific activities and free-in-air neutron doses (13).

B) Gamma rays

When thermoluminescent materials are exposed to ionizing radiations, some of the free electrons are trapped at lattice imperfections in the crystalline solid. They remain trapped for long periods at ambient temperatures. If the temperature is increased, electrons are thermally released from the traps and light is emitted as they recombine with oppositely charged centers. The quantity of light emitted can be proportional to the absorbed energy in the material. Bricks and tiles can be utilized as thermoluminescent materials (5).

The thermoluminescent yield of bricks and ornamental tiles was measured with a handmade apparatus. The gamma ray dose of the A-bombs was estimated from the results of the thermoluminescent measurements, using a gamma ray source spectrally equivalent to the A-bombs prepared by X-rays from a 6 MeV linear accelerator for a high energy component and gamma rays from ^{60}Co and ^{137}Cs for a medium energy component. Table III gives the results of the thermoluminescent measurements and resultant free-in-air gamma ray doses (15).

C) *Kyoto University*

A group at Kyoto University (15) has estimated free-in-air gamma ray doses with thermoluminescent measurements of roof tiles.

6. *Free-in-air doses of T65D*

The precision (coefficient of variation) of NIRS dose estimates was estimated to be less than 0.11 for gamma rays and less than 0.15 for neutrons. NIRS doses as compared with York's values shown in Fig. 3 provided only a minor difference for gamma rays and agreed with that for neutrons in Nagasaki, but a large difference of approximately 50% for neutrons and 30%–70% for gamma rays at distances of 500–1,500 m from ground zero in Hiroshima. Auxier and his co-workers (4) estimated the percent probable error in their dose estimates. Because of the uncertainties which persist concerning the yield of the Hiroshima bomb, the error in the Hiroshima estimates was considered to be about 30%. The doses for Nagasaki were estimated to be accurate to within about 10%.

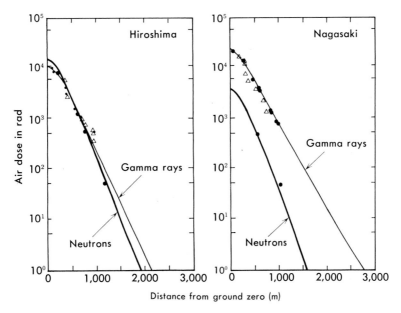

FIG. 4. T65D free-in-air doses for ORNL and Japanese data, Hiroshima and Nagasaki. ═, ORNL; •●, NIRS; △, Kyoto University.

The free-in-air doses of gamma rays and neutrons determined by *in situ* measurements by two Japanese groups agreed with the ORNL values estimated as a result of Operation BREN (Fig. 4), although there is some scatter. Milton and Shohoji (*24*) have described the T65D system of dose estimates in Hiroshima and Nagasaki. They proposed the free-in-air dose curves calculated from the parameters given by Auxier *et al.* (*4*) in the T65D system.

7. *Nine parameters*

Gamma rays and neutrons differ in their penetration, and shielding materials in their penetrability. For survivors in the open unshielded on all sides, the best estimates of the dose received are free-in-air doses. However, survivors shielded on one side by a heavy wall received the full free-in-air dose less some fraction screened out by the wall. The survivors exposed in a house received only a small fraction of the free-in-air dose at a corresponding distance, depending on numerous characteristics of the shielding configuration. The ORNL group developed a technique of globe operation to evaluate transmission values for these shielding situations. The globe consisted of a sphere of transparent plastic with latitude and longitude lines inscribed on the surface at 10° intervals and a small bulb approximating a point source of light at the center. When placed in a scale model of the shielding configuration so that its center represents the survivor of interest, the axis was pointed in the direction of the radiation source, and its projection on portions of the model showed what part of the incident radiation was intercepted by the shield. Using the experimentally determined angular distribution function of radiations from the A-bomb tests in conjunction with the measurements made with the globe operation, the fraction of intercepted radiations was determined. The dose at the point of interest, D, was calculated by the following equation:

$$D = (TF_1 + F_2)D_{air} \qquad (2)$$

where F_1 is the fraction of radiation intercepted, T is the transmission rate of the shield, F_2 is the fraction of total radiation which is not blocked, and D_{air} is the free-in-air dose at the location.

In addition to the globe operation, the ORNL group developed a more sophisticated nine parameter procedure to estimate the transmission rates to be applied to the free-in-air dose for the evaluations of the dose for survivors exposed in typical Japanese houses. The nine parameters for gamma rays and neutrons were 1) floor number, 2) slant penetration distance of direct radiation through the house, 3) number of interior walls shielding the survivors from the front, 4) number of interior walls shielding the survivor from the side, 5) presence of a shielding structure in front, 6) size of the shielding structure in front, if present, 7) presence of a lateral shielding structure, 8) distance from any unshielded window in the direction of the burst point, and 9) height above the air/ground interface. Using these parameters, the radiation dose at the point of interest was calculated by the following equation:
Neutrons:

$$D_n = [A_1 \exp{(-G_1)} + A_2 G_2 + A_3 G_3 + A_4 G_4 + A_5 G_5 + A_6 \exp{(-G_6)} + A_8 G_8 + A_8]D_{air} \qquad (3)$$

Gamma rays:

$$D_\gamma = [A_1 A_2 \exp{(-G)} + A_2 \exp{(-G_1)} + A_4 G_3 + A_5 G_4 + A_6 G_5 + A_7 G_6]D_{air} \qquad (4)$$

TABLE IV. BREN Average Gamma Ray Transmission Factors for
a Single-story House in Hiroshima

Event	Neutron	Gamma ray
Plumbbob	0.507 ± 0.11	0.769 ± 0.11
Hardtack	0.407 ± 0.09	0.952 ± 0.15
BREN reactor	0.151 ± 0.15	1.35 ± 0.08
BREN ^{60}Co		0.464 ± 0.18

where D_n represents neutron dose and D_γ gamma ray dose in Japanese houses or other structures. A_i is the constant and G_i is a geometrical factor related to the nine parameters. The ratios of D_n/D_{air} and D_γ/D_{air} represent the transmission factor for neutrons and gamma rays, respectively. The BREN average gamma ray transmission factors for a single house at Hiroshima and Nagasaki are given in Table IV. These numbers are based on the single house experiment with the HPRR and ^{60}Co gamma ray source. The effect of surrounding houses on the transmission factor (1) was assumed to change the single house value by a power of 2 and 3/2, respectively.

In the dose determinations for survivors in the LSS, organ or tissue doses should be evaluated using the house transmission factors and dose distributions of A-bomb radiation in the body of the survivor. The NIRS and ORNL groups have determined some conversion factors from free-in-air doses to organ or tissue doses for the organ dosimetry (9–12, 16).

To evaluate the late biological effects of the A-bombs a primary requirement is the most precise knowledge concerning not only the exposure to the initial radiations of the bombs but the exposure to secondary radiations from residual radiations released from neutron-induced radioactivity and fission products on the ground and medical exposure before and after the time of bombs. The latter doses have been evaluated by some authors (8, 25, 33).

Recent Reassessments of A-Bomb Radiation Dosimetry

There are significant differences in the biological effects on the survivors in Hiroshima and Nagasaki. In the T65D system, these differences appeared to be explained by the existence of a significant neutron dose in Hiroshima as compared with the dose in Nagasaki. Milton and Shohoji (24) predicted that the T65D estimates were not final and should be revised immediately when new information became available. A-bomb dose depends on many factors, such as the design of the bomb, the TNT equivalent yield, the height above the ground at which the bomb explodes, the density and humidity of the air, and numerous other factors. Information on source terms such as spectra and intensities of radiation sources is very important for the dose estimations of survivors after an explosion of an A-bomb and even after a critical accident in nuclear facilities.

The first modern calculations of the output spectra of neutrons and gamma rays from the A-bombs exploded over Hiroshima and Nagasaki were declassified by the US Department of Energy (DOE) in 1976 and were distributed as a letter (36) which was used in recent reassessments of A-bomb doses. The ORNL (17) and LLNL (20) groups recalculated the free-in-air doses of gamma rays and neutrons on the basis of the output spectra calculated by Preeg, using a computer code employing "discrete ordinate transport" (DOT) techniques. Components on which they recalculated the dose

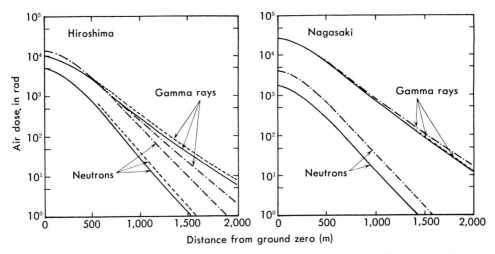

FIG. 5. Revised free-in-air doses by ORNL (*17*) and LLNL (*20*), Hiroshima and Nagasaki. –·–, T65D; ——, ORNL; – – – –, LLNL.

TABLE V. Differences of Dose Determination between LLNL and ORNL

Parameter	LLNL	ORNL
Source terms	Preeg-LANL	Preeg-LANL
Transport calculation	DOT technique-ORNL	DOT technique-ORNL
Cross-section	ENDL	ENDF/B-IV and V
Atmosphere (ground-burst height)	Homogeneous	Tiered with decreasing density of air with height
Ground composition	4 elements (H, O, Si, and Al)	(H, O, Si, and Al)
Height of burst	Hiroshima, 570 m	Hiroshima, 580 m
	Nagasaki, 503 m	Nagasaki, 503 m
Yield of bomb	Hiroshima, 15 kton	Hiroshima, 12.5 kton
	Nagasaki, 22 kton	Nagasaki, 22 kton
Delayed gamma ray calculation code	ITTRI (1964) (semi-experimental)	NUIDEA (1981) (theoretical)

consisted of 1) prompt gamma rays and neutrons from bomb leakage directly out of the weapon, 2) secondary component of gamma rays resulting from neutron interactions with atmospheric nitrogen, and 3) gamma rays from the debris cloud of a nuclear explosion. Their results are shown in Fig. 5. The data do not completely agree with each other because they used some different factors and some different assumptions in their dose calculations (Table V). As shown in Fig. 5, the neutron dose in Hiroshima was much less than the T65D estimates by factors varying from about 4 at a ground distance of 1,000 m to 8 at 2,000 m, and the gamma ray doses were greater than the T65D estimates starting at a ground distance of about 1,000 m and were probably larger by a factor of about 3 at 2,000 m. In Nagasaki, the situation was reversed with respect to gamma rays, and the T65D estimates were higher, but the differences were small, for example, about 20% at a ground distance of 1,000 m and 30% at 2,000 m. Although these results are preliminary, the T65D estimates must be revised on the basis of new information such as leakage output radiation spectra from the A-bombs.

The neutron and gamma ray doses received by the survivors in Hiroshima and Nagasaki must be accurate within some limits if conclusions drawn from studies of the

the current T65D estimates take into account distance from ground zero and shielding by surrounding structures. Since, however, the organ or tissue doses depend on the orientation of the survivor at the time of explosion, it must be known whether the individual was facing toward the bomb or away from it. The uncertainties in information on the orientation and the posture of each survivor can make large differences in the evaluation of the relationship between corresponding organ or tissue dose and the stochastic effect resulting from the epidemiological survey of survivors in Hiroshima and Nagasaki, even if the physical parameters to assign dose to survivors were measured with a high accuracy. Woolson *et al.* are developing a dosimetric system for the survivors including organ or tissue dose (*40*).

CONCLUSION

Since 1980, many discussions concerning the reevaluation of A-bomb dose in Hiroshima and Nagasaki have taken place among US and Japanese specialists, mostly in the field of nuclear and radiation physics and radiobiology. However, no conclusion has been reached to date, even for the source terms of the Hiroshima bomb. A comparison of calculated radiation doses with experimental *in situ* measurements in Japan is extremely desirable as a rationale for acceptance of reevaluated doses. After this, the US and Japanese committee on the reevaluation of A-bomb doses must decide on a single dosimetric parameter which should be used for the determination of a survivor's dose in further epidemiological surveys at RERF. At the second US-Japan Joint Workshop for Reassessment of A-bomb Radiation Dosimetry held in 1983 in Hiroshima, special subgroups were formed to discuss and report on the following subjects, in order to derive some conclusions of radiation dose estimates as soon as possible: 1) A-bomb yields, 2) source terms, 3) radiation transport in air, 4) thermoluminescent dosimetry, 5) neutron activation and neutron dosimetry, 6) fallout and induced radioactivity, 7) house shielding, 8) self shielding (organ or tissue dosimetry), and 9) uncertainties.

It is expected that DS86 (Dosimetric System, 1986) will be available in June 1986. A tentative epidemiological survey may be undertaken during December 1986.

The recently revised doses for neutrons were much lower than the T65 neutron dose in both cities. For gamma rays in Hiroshima, the revised doses are higher than the T65D, and in Nagasaki the revised doses were almost the same as the T65D. The ratio of neutron dose to gamma ray dose in Hiroshima was still higher than in Nagasaki. For example, neutron dose at 1,000 m from ground zero was about 30 rad in Hiroshima and about 13 rad in Nagasaki. Gamma ray dose at the same distance was about 300 rad in Hiroshima and about 750 rad in Nagasaki. The ratio of neutron dose to gamma ray dose decreased rapidly with increasing distance from ground zero. The neutron component in Hiroshima was significantly higher at a short distance from ground zero as compared with that in Nagasaki. On the other hand, the transmission factors of typical Japanese houses recently proposed can reduce the gamma ray doses of survivors by a factor of 2. According to the neutron spectrum on the ground level recently calculated by Pace (unpublished), the lower energy part of neutrons was predominant. As recent calculations by Kaul (unpublished) indicate, for the significantly degraded spectrum of neutrons in Hiroshima, the neutron capture (n, γ) component and (n, p) component from nitrogen capture will become more important and, when these neutron capture components are added in recoil ions from elastic collisions, the total absorbed organ dose of neutrons is higher than the free-in-air dose by several orders of magnitude at very low energies of neutrons. As a result, it appears that leukemia and other disease incidences at lower exposure levels in Hiroshima may be due to gamma rays rather than neutrons. However, this may not be true at higher exposure levels in Hiroshima. Recent reevaluations of A-bomb doses can lead to lower neutron doses compared with the T65D, but for risk estimates of gamma rays, the recently revised doses may bring more reasonable values than before. In any case, a reanalysis of data on biological effects among the A-bomb survivors should be regarded as highly tentative and speculative until some dosimetric parameters have been investigated in more detail.

REFERENCES

1. Auxier, J. A. Attenuation of weapons radiation; Application to Japanese houses, operation Hardtack. USAEC Report WT-1725, Oak Ridge National Laboratory, NTIS (1960).
2. Auxier, J. A. Technical Concept—Operation BREN, USAEC Rep. CEX-62.01, NTIS (1962).
3. Auxier, J. A. Ichiban, Radiation Dosimetry for the Survivors of the Bombings of Hiroshima and Nagasaki, ERDA Critical Review Series, YID-27080, NTIS (1977).
4. Auxier, J. A., Cheka, J. S., Haywood, F. F., Jones, T. D., and Thorngate, J. H. Free-field-radiation dose distributions from the Hiroshima and Nagasaki bombings. *Health Phys.*, **12**, 425–429 (1966).
5. Daniels, F., and Saunders, D. F. The thermoluminescence of rocks. *Science*, **111**, 461–462 (1950).
6. Glasstone, S. The Effects of Nuclear Weapons, US Atomic Energy Commission (1957).
7. Hamada, T. Measurement of ^{32}P activity induced in sulfur in Hiroshima. *In* "US-Japan Joint Workshop for Reassessment of A-bomb Dosimetry," ed. D. J. Thompson, pp. 45–56 (1983). RERF, Hiroshima.
8. Hashizume, T., Maruyama, T., Kumamoto, Y., Kato, Y., and Kawamura, S. Estimation of gamma-ray dose from neutron-induced radioactivity in Hiroshima and Nagasaki. *Health Phys.*, **17**, 761–771 (1969).
9. Hashizume, T., Maruyama, T., Nishizawa, K., and Nishimura, A. Dose estimation of human fetus exposed in utero to radiations from atomic bombs in Hiroshima and Nagasaki. *J. Radiat. Res.*, **14**, 346–362 (1973).
10. Hashizume, T., Maruyama, T., Nishizawa, K., and Nishimura, A. Estimation of absorbed dose in thyroids and gonads of survivors in Hiroshima and Nagasaki. *Acta Radiologaica*, **13**, 411–424 (1974).
11. Hashizume, T., Maruyama, T., Nishizawa, K., and Fukuhisa, K. Mean bone marrow dose of atomic bomb survivors in Hiroshima and Nagasaki. *J. Radiat. Res.*, **18**, 67–83 (1977).
12. Hashizume, T., Maruyama, T., Nishizawa, K., Noda, Y., Fukuhisa, K., and Takeda, E. Determinations of organ or tissue doses to survivors in Hiroshima and Nagasaki. *J. Radiat. Res.*, **21**, 213–230 (1980).
13. Hashizume, T., Maruyama, T., Shiragai, A., Tanaka, E., Izawa, M., Kawamura, S., and Nagaoka, S. Estimation of the air dose from the atomic bombs in Hiroshima and Nagasaki. *Health Phys.*, **13**, 149–161 (1967).
14. Hurst, G. S. and Ritchie, R. H. Fast neutron dosimetry. *Radiology*, **60**, 864–869 (1953).
15. Ichikawa, Y., Higashimura, T., and Sidei, T. Thermoluminescence dosimetry of gamma rays from atomic bombs in Hiroshima and Nagasaki. *Health Phys.*, **12**, 395–405 (1966).
16. Kerr, G. D. Organ dose estimates for the Japanese atomic bomb survivors. *Health Phys.*, **37**, 487–508 (1979).
17. Kerr, G. D. Review of dosimetry for the atomic bomb survivors, Proc. 4th Symp. on

Neutron Dosimetry, Munich-Neuherberg, Federal Republic of Germany, Vol. 1, pp. 501–513 (1981).

18. Kerr, G. D. Findings of a recent Oak Ridge National Laboratory review of dosimetry for the Japanese atomic-bomb survivors, Proc. Symp. at Germantown, Technical Information Center US Department of Energy, pp. 52–97 (1982).

19. Kerr, G. D., Pace, J. V. III, and Scott, W. H. Tissue kerma *vs.* distance relationship for initial nuclear radiation from the atomic bombs Hiroshima and Nagasaki, Proc. A-bomb Dosimetry Workshop, Nagasaki, pp. 57–103 (1983).

20. Loewe, W. E. and Mendelsohn, E. Revised estimates of dose at Hiroshima and Nagasaki, and possible consequences for radiation induced leukemia (preliminary). Tech. Rep., D-80-14 (1980).

21. Malik, J. Yields of the Hiroshima and Nagasaki explosions, Proc. Symp. Germantown, DOE Symp. Ser. 55, USDOE, pp. 98–110 (1982).

22. Maruyama, T., Kumamoto, Y., Noda, Y., Yamada, H., Okamoto, Y., Fujita, S., and Hashizume, T. Reassessment of gamma-ray dose estimates from thermoluminescent yields in Hiroshima and Nagasaki, Proc. A-bomb Dosimetry Workshop, Nagasaki, pp. 122–137 (1983).

23. Maruyama, T., Kumamoto, Y., Noda, Y., Iwai, K., and Michikawa, T. Shielding parameters and standard Japanese for organ dosimetry. *In* "Second US-Japan Workshop for Reassessment of A-bomb Dosimetry," pp. 64–66 (1983). RERF, Hiroshima.

24. Milton, R. C. and Shohoji, T. Tentative 1965 radiation dose estimation for atomic bomb survivors. ABCC Tech. Rep. 1-68 (1968).

25. Okajima, S. Dose estimation from residual and fallout radioactivity; fallout in the Nagasaki Nishiyama District. *J. Radiat. Res.* (Suppl.) 16, 35–41 (1975).

26. Okajima, S. and Miyajima, J. Measurement of neutron-induced ^{152}Eu radioactivity in Nagasaki, Proc. A-bomb Dosimetry Workshop, Nagasaki, pp. 156–168 (1983).

27. RERF: Second US-Japan Joint Workshop for Reassessment of Atomic Bomb Radiation Dosimetry in Hiroshima and Nagasaki, Proceedings of a Workshop Held at Hiroshima (1983).

28. Ritchie, R. H., and Hurst, G. S. Penetration of weapons radiation; Application to the Hiroshima-Nagasaki studies. *Health Phys.*, 1, 390–404 (1959).

29. Scott, W. H. Delayed radiation at Hiroshima and Nagasaki, Proc. Symp. at Germantown, Technical Information Center US Department of Energy, pp. 159–178 (1983).

30. Sinclair, W. K. and Failla, P. Dosimetry of the atomic bomb survivors. *Radiat. Res.*, 88, 437–447 (1981).

31. Sinclair, W. K. and Sakanoue, M. Rapporteur's report, Proc. 2nd A-bomb Dosimetry Workshop at Hiroshima, pp. 59–63 (1983).

32. Tajima, E. Estimation of the Hiroshima bomb yield and weather conditions at the time of the bomb, Proc. 2nd A-bomb Dosimetry Workshop, Hiroshima, pp. 1–13 (1983).

33. Takeshita, K. Dose estimation from residual and fallout radioactivity; area surveys. *J. Radiat. Res.* (Suppl.), 16, 24–31 (1975).

34. USDOE. Reevaluations of Dosimetric Factors Hiroshima and Nagasaki, Proceedings of a symposium held at Germantown, Technical Information Center US Department of Energy, ed. Bond, V. P. and Thiessen, J. W. (1982).

35. Wagner, E. G. and Hurst, G. S. A G-M tube X-ray dosimeter with low neutron sensitivity. *Health Phys.*, 5, 20–26 (1961).

36. Whalen, P. P. Status of Los Alamos efforts related to Hiroshima and Nagasaki dose estimates, Germantown, DOE Symp. Ser. 55, US DOE, pp. 111–130 (1982).

37. Whalen, P. P. Source terms for the initial radiations, Proc. A-bomb Dosimetry Workshop, Nagasaki, pp. 13–44 (1983).

38. Whalen, P. P., Soran, P. D., Malenfant, R., and Forehand, H. M., Jr. Experiments at Los

Alamos National Laboratory with the Replica of Hiroshima Weapon, Proc. 2nd A-bomb Dosimetry Workshop, Hiroshima, pp. 21–15 (1983).

39. Woolson, W. A. personal communication (1984).

40. Woolson, W. A. Gritzner, M. L., and Egbert, S. D. Coupled houseman shielding calculations for atomic bomb survivors organ dosimetry, Proc. Workshop, 2nd A-bomb Dosimetry Workshop, Hiroshima, pp. 72–75 (1982).

41. Woolson, W. A., Marcum, J., Scott, W. H., and Staggs, V. E. Building transmission factors, Proc. Symp. at Germantown, Technical Information Center US Department of Energy, pp. 179–208 (1982).

42. Yamazaki, F. and Sugimoto, A. Radioactive phosphorous ^{32}P in human bone and sulfur insulators in Hiroshima, Collection of Investigative Reports on Atomic Bomb Disaster, Vol. I, pp. 16–18 (1953). Japanese Science Promotion Society, Tokyo.

TUMOR AND TISSUE REGISTRIES IN
HIROSHIMA AND NAGASAKI

Tetsuo MONZEN*1 and Toshiro WAKABAYASHI*2

Department of Pathology, Hiroshima Prefectural Hospital,[1] *and*
Department of Epidemiology and Statistics[2],
Radiation Effects Research Foundation

Continued monitoring of tumor incidence is an important part of the surveillance of health effects of atomic bomb (A-bomb) radiation. The Radiation Effects Research Foundation (RERF) (formerly Atomic Bomb Casualty Commission (ABCC)) has been engaged in the operation of tumor and tissue registries in Hiroshima and Nagasaki. These registries have been instrumental in studying risk of various specific cancer sites (thyroid, breast, lung, stomach, colorectal, and salivary gland) in a defined sample of A-bomb survivors. A recent analysis of registry data revealed little basis for suspecting systematic biases of registry data (*e.g.*, hospital-related, or diagnostic biases related to radiation dose) which may confound observed association of cancer and radiation. The analysis also showed similarities in relative risk of cancer based on incidence and mortality data. However, absolute risks estimated from mortality data may underestimate the true magnitude for certain cancer sites (including breast, stomach, lung, and uterus). The registry data are also useful in assessing secular trends of radiation-induced cancer incidence which are essential in determining the latency of cancer.

The Atomic Bomb Casualty Commission (ABCC) and its successor, the Radiation Effects Research Foundation (RERF), have been engaged in the operation of tumor registries for the last 20 years and tissue registries for the last 10 years in Hiroshima and Nagasaki under the entrustment of local medical associations. These registries have served as important data sources in assessment of cancer incidence in the RERF sample of persons exposed to atomic bomb (A-bomb) radiation as well as geographically defined populations. Incidence data offer an advantage over mortality data in that the former provide a direct measure of cancer risk. This is particularly important when dealing with tumors associated with relatively low mortality such as thyroid and breast cancer. Also, detailed diagnostic information gathered from medical records can enhance accuracy of diagnosis. The significance of detailed diagnostic information is increased with the recent decline in autopsy rates.

Activities of the tumor registries in the early years were described in several publications (*5, 6, 8*). Later the tumor and tissue registry data have been used extensively at RERF for epidemiologic and pathologic studies of specific cancer cites in relation to A-bomb radiation exposure. These sites include thyroid, breast, lung, stomach, colorectal,

---

*1 Ujina Kanda 1-5, Minami-ku, Hiroshima 730, Japan (門前徹夫).
*2 Hijiyama Park 5-2, Minami-ku, Hiroshima 732, Japan (若林俊郎).

and salivary gland (2, 12–14, 16, 18, 19, 22, 23). Overall analysis of the latest tumor incidence data of the Life Span Study (LSS) sample in Nagasaki (for the period 1959–78) has been published (17). Recently analysis has been made of the updated Hiroshima registry data and the findings of this analysis are to be published.

Tumor Registry

Agreements were exchanged between ABCC and the City Medical Associations of Hiroshima and Nagasaki for the initiation of Tumor Registries in Hiroshima in 1957 and in Nagasaki in 1958. The City Medical Associations of the two cities have organized the Tumor Statistics Committee which is responsible for the maintenance of the Registry and registration of tumor cases, while ABCC (and later RERF) provided technical support. At the outset, registration was quite active as described in several reports (5, 6, 8). It became less active in subsequent years, especially in Hiroshima, mainly because of difficulty in securing collaboration from large hospitals. However, through concentrated efforts during the past few years in updating data collection, the Hiroshima registry data now appear to merit analysis.

For registries to be effective, all tumor cases should be ascertained. While cases with histologically confirmed neoplasms are ideal for diagnostic accuracy, they may represent a small and possibly selected portion of tumor cases. The Hiroshima and Nagasaki registries, like most other registries, assemble information from various data sources (clinical, pathological, radiological, *etc.*).

As a rule the examining physician is requested to submit a report whenever a case is detected. A notification card in a sealed envelope is used for preservation of confidentiality and privacy. Major hospitals are also requested to submit their reports once a month. As the burden of assigned physicians at these major hospitals is heavy, and the assignment is often rotated among the physicians, the number of reports submitted is not always constant. Cases reported by physicians (private or at hospitals) make up only a small proportion of all registered patients (10% in Hiroshima and 3% in Nagasaki).

Most cases (79% in Hiroshima and 85% in Nagasaki) are ascertained by screening of hospitalized tumor cases undertaken by trained RERF field personnel. They search autopsy protocols, clinical and pathological reports, as well as surgical operation records. At surgery, tumors can be confirmed directly, and with recent progress in operative techniques, surgical records are an especially useful source of data on nonfatal cancers (*e.g.*, breast, uterine cervix, and urinary bladder). X-ray diagnoses and clinical examinations are still important sources of data, and diagnosis by cytologic and endoscopic examination has recently increased. The latter should be classified separately, but the number of cases is still small and therefore is included in the clinical diagnosis category. When information obtained from these various sources is checked against death certificates, many tumors are found for which no hospital record has been obtained. Thus, death certificates remain an important source of ascertainment, accounting for 11% of all cases in Hiroshima and 12% in Nagasaki.

Registered tumors are all malignant neoplasms plus benign neoplasms of the brain, salivary gland, and colon. Polyposis of the stomach and digestive organs is also included. Information is gathered on name, sex, date of birth, present address, tumor diagnosed, method and date of diagnosis, date of death and medical institution, and clinic or physician. Information obtained is checked against the Master File to determine whether it

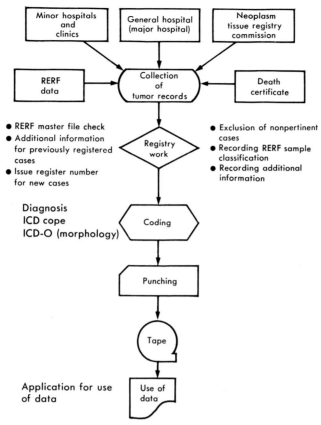

FIG. 1. Flow chart, Tumor Registry.

is a new or registered case. After determining the validity of registration, a code is assigned based on the International Classification of Diseases (ICD) 9th revision (21) and the data are stored on magnetic tapes (Fig. 1).

Multiple reports of the same tumor sometimes occur. There are cases in which the same cancer is reported by different hospitals, at different periods, with diagnosis based on different diagnostic methods. When this occurs, a report using the best available information is coded and filed. Among the alternative methods of ascertainment, autopsy findings take precedence followed by surgical pathological statements, surgical findings, radiography, clinical examinations, and finally the statement as to cause of death recorded on the death certificate.

Among the clinically diagnosed cases are those which the attending physician labeled possible cancer (e.g., possible cancer of the stomach or possible pancreatic cancer). The qualification "possible" is maintained in the computer record so that analysis can be made excluding these cases, if desired. It has been suggested that overregistration may have occurred due to inclusion of possible cancer and occult cancer (recognized only at autopsy) in the Hiroshima and Nagasaki data. The proportion of possible cancer cases among total cases is 8.6% in Hiroshima and 12.6% in Nagasaki. They are relatively less frequent in Hiroshima than in Nagasaki and their contribution to overregistration is less in Hiroshima. The mean frequency of autopsy among deaths occurring in the LSS sample during 1961–75, which is the major source of detecting occult cancer, is 31%

in Hiroshima and 30% in Nagasaki, so it is likely that occult cancer influences the two
registries in a similar way.

    If a patient is registered with multiple tumor sites, it is difficult to determine whether
they are single or multiple primary tumors, particularly on the basis of the limited clinical
and pathologic information available. In our tumor registries, multiple cancers are
registered whenever a case of multiple primary cancer is suspected, and such cases are
reviewed using the guidelines on cancer registration published by the International
Agency for Research on Cancer (*11*). In Hiroshima 204 (3%) of 6,608 reviewed cases
were considered to have multiple primary cancer and in Nagasaki, 46 (2%) of 1,870
cases were regarded as multiple primary cancer.

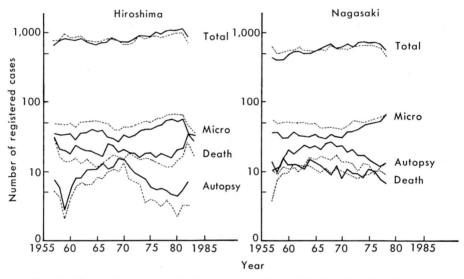

Fig. 2. Tumor Registry activities by city, sex, and year. Total number of registered
cases. Rates for autopsies, microscopically confirmed cases, and death certificate
only cases. ———, male; ----, female.

TABLE I.   Average Annual Incidence Rate (per 100,000) in Hiroshima
City, Nagasaki City, and Japan

City	Sex	Year		
		1975–77	1976–78	1977–79
Hiroshima	Male	223.6	236.5	239.6
	Female	164.6	162.2	162.3
Nagasaki	Male	250.4	252.6	257.6
	Female	184.6	178.8	175.9
		1976	1977	1978
Japan (estimates)	Male	203.3	206.1	209.4
	Female	136.0	137.9	138.5

Age-adjusted to world population.

    Estimated incidence for Japan is obtained from Cancer Incidence in Japan 1975–79 (*4*). Hiroshima in-
cidence rates are based on RERF's most recent estimates.

Data are routinely tabulated by site, age, and hospital, and the tabulations are distributed to each cooperative hospital in Hiroshima as feedback material. Stored information has been used at RERF for studies of several specific cancer sites. Comparative incidence studies among several tumor registries have also been conducted in cooperation with the cancer research group based on research funds from the Ministry of Health and Welfare.

Figure 2 presents the registered cases over the years in Hiroshima and Nagasaki by different ascertainment methods. The proportion of cases identified from death certificates alone has been relatively low, especially in Nagasaki. Table I shows the cancer incidence rate generated from the Hiroshima and Nagasaki registry data. Compared with the average cancer incidence rate for other prefectural registries in Japan, the age-adjusted incidence rates for all sites in both Hiroshima and Nagasaki are slightly higher. Several reasons for this are possible, including 1) the completeness of reports resulting from active data collection utilizing field personnel as compared to voluntary reporting by other registries; 2) overregistration because of the inclusion of doubtful diagnosis and occult cancer in the Hiroshima and Nagasaki registries; and 3) the high incidence of cancer in Hiroshima and Nagasaki.

Tissue Registry

In 1973, the Hiroshima Prefectural Medical Association initiated a Tissue Registry for registering surgical and pathological specimens of tumor tissues. The significance of this program lies in the collection of tumor cases based on tissue diagnosis and their reproducibility. Financial support was provided for three years from the US National Institutes of Health-National Cancer Institute to the Hiroshima Prefectural Medical Association *via* ABCC. With this support, the Medical Association organized the Hiroshima Prefectural Tissue Registry Committee and established its Registration Office at the Medical Association Hall. The registry is operated by a working committee composed of pathologists engaged in histological diagnosis at principal medical institutions, epidemiologists, statisticians, and representatives from the Leukemia Registry.

The Registration Office headed by an experienced pathologist requests the pathologist-in-charge at each medical institution to submit one H & E-stained tissue slide, a copy of the pathological diagnosis made at the institution, and a copy of the pathology examination request forwarded from clinical departments. For each reported case, a part-time pathologist reviews slides and assigns ICD-Oncology Codes (20).

In Hiroshima, approximately 14,000 tissue slides are submitted yearly, and approximately 10,000 cases are finally registered. The ratio of malignant cases to benign cases is about 3 to 2. In males, this ratio is 3 to 1, but it is higher in females due to benign tumors of the uterus, ovary, and breast.

The Tissue Registry in Nagasaki was begun in 1974, a year after the initiation of the Hiroshima Tissue Registry. Funding and establishment conditions were similar to those in Hiroshima. The Nagasaki Tissue Registry is conducted by the City Medical Association, which organized the Nagasaki Neoplasm Tissue Registry Commission and established the Registration Office in the Department of Pathology, Nagasaki University School of Medicine. The geographic area covered includes Nagasaki City and three adjacent cities and their suburbs. Different from the Hiroshima registry, tissue blocks are collected along with brief clinical records. Four specimens are prepared from each block at the Tissue Registry Laboratory and they are reviewed by four pathologists on the Pathology Expert Committee. If an agreement cannot be reached on diagnosis, the slides are submitted for review at a later date. The Manual of Tumor Nomenclature and Coding is employed for coding (1).

Analysis of Incidence Data

Data accumulated in the Tumor Registries have been found invaluable in assessing the carcinogenic role of radiation. Almost all of the original data for RERF cancer studies (including thyroid, breast, lung, stomach, colorectal, and salivary gland) are based on data from the Tumor and Tissue Registries. Overall analysis of Tumor Registry data in both cities has recently been completed for the period 1959–78, and some of the findings from this analysis are presented.

Subjects included in the analysis are members of the LSS extended sample in Nagasaki and alive as of January 1959. There are 17,936 persons in the sample, constituting a total of 319,803 person-years at risk during the observation period 1959–78. The dosimetry used is based on a revision of the original T65 dose system (T65DR), which takes into account the recently relocated Nagasaki ground zero point (10) and a standardization of the rounding process in calculating individual dose (15).

1. Potential sources of bias

Several potential sources of bias in the registry data may lead to spuriously increased cancer incidence in high radiation dose groups compared with low radiation or control groups. For example, biases related to radiation dose may originate in hospitals from which registry data were obtained. However, the distribution of registered tumor

TABLE II.   Number of All Cancer Sites by Hospital and Exposure Status, Nagasaki, 1959–78

Hospital	T65 revised kerma dose in rad						NIC[a]	Unknown
	Total	0	1–9	10–49	50–99	100+		
Total	1,412	274	455	262	107	314	404	54
	100.0%	19.4%	32.2%	18.6%	7.6%	22.2%		
ABCC/RERF	520	103	153	96	45	123	156	20
	100.0	19.8	29.4	18.5	8.6	23.7		
Nagasaki University	347	61	116	61	28	81	91	18
	100.0	17.6	33.4	17.6	8.1	23.3		
Citizens hospital	78	17	25	17	5	14	35	2
	100.0	21.8	32.1	21.8	6.4	17.9		
A-bomb hospital	207	40	73	36	9	49	19	8
	100.0	19.3	35.3	17.4	4.3	23.7		
Other large hospitals	128	28	36	28	11	25	35	4
	100.0	21.9	28.1	21.9	8.6	19.5		
Practitioners (private)	79	13	32	16	7	11	35	2
	100.0	16.5	40.5	20.2	8.9	13.9		
Other	53	12	20	8	2	11	33	0
	100.0	22.6	37.7	15.1	3.8	20.8		

[a] Not in the city.

Difference in distribution by hospital among five exposed groups (NIC and Unknown excluded). Not significant. $\chi^2 = 18.46$, $d.f. = 24$, $p = 0.78$.

TABLE III. Number of All Cancer Sites by Method of Ascertainment and
Exposure Status, Nagasaki, 1959–78

	T65 revised kerma dose in rad						NIC[a]	Unknown
	Total	0	1–9	10–49	50–99	100+		
Total	1,412	274	455	262	107	314	404	54
	100.0%	100.0%	100.0%	100.0%	100.0%	100.0%		
a) Confirmed	1,015	186	335	188	85	221	273	37
	71.9	67.9	73.6	71.8	79.4	70.4		
1. Autopsy	420	76	140	82	40	82	114	19
	29.7	27.8	30.8	31.3	37.4	26.1		
2. Surgical	514	96	164	89	36	129	136	15
	36.4	35.0	36.0	34.0	33.6	41.1		
3. Operation	81	14	31	17	9	10	23	3
	5.7	5.1	6.8	6.5	8.4	3.2		
b) Other	397	88	120	74	22	93	131	17
	28.1	32.1	26.4	28.2	20.6	29.6		
4. Radiography	129	34	37	25	6	27	35	7
	9.1	12.4	8.1	9.5	5.6	8.6		
5. Clinical	173	36	48	32	9	48	42	8
	12.3	13.1	10.6	12.2	8.4	15.3		
6. Death certificate	95	18	35	17	7	18	54	2
	6.7	6.6	7.7	6.5	6.6	5.7		

[a] Not in the city.

Difference in distribution by six methods of ascertainment is not significant among five exposure groups (NIC and Unknown excluded). $\chi^2 = 24.54$, $d.f. = 20$, $p = 0.22$.

Difference in distribution by Confirmed and Other is not significant among five exposure groups (NIC and Unknown excluded). $\chi^2 = 6.2$, $d.f. = 4$, $p = 0.18$.

cases by radiation dose did not differ among hospitals (Table II). Knowledge of dose on the part of the physician and/or survivor may result in frequent use of certain diagnostic techniques (e.g., surgical pathology) or infrequent use of other methods (e.g., radiography) among A-bomb survivors. However, data in Table III show no consistent pattern for preferred diagnostic methods by dose group. The highest dose group (100+ rad) had fewer cases undergoing autopsy and more cases subjected to pathologic examination, but the difference was not statistically significant. Cases confirmed by autopsy, surgical pathology, or surgery accounted for 72% of all cases, and the proportion of confirmed cases did not differ by dose group. Based on these findings there is little evidence to suspect the presence of systematic biases in the registry data.

Another source of potential bias is differential migration for different dose groups. Separate analysis of data from a subset of the LSS failed to disclose differential rates of migration for various dose groups or by time period (3). More recently, other evidence on this issue has become available as a result of a mail survey of exposed LSS members. These data, too, fail to reveal systematic differences in migration by dose and time which could obscure a radiation effect on cancer incidence or create a spurious one.

2. Cancer risk and radiation exposure

Table IV presents the relative risk for all and selected sites of cancer for the 100+ rad group (vs. 0–9 or 0 rad groups), using three sources of ascertainment: all sources (all); autopsy, pathology, and surgery reports (confirmed); and death certificates (mor-

TABLE IV.   Relative Risk (100+*vs.* 0–9 rad) of All and Selected Cancer
by Method of Ascertainment: Nagasaki, 1959–78

Site	Source		
	All sources	Confirmed	Mortality
All sites[a]	1.70 (1.48 1.95)	1.76 (1.49 2.07)	1.29 (1.05 1.56)
Leukemia	3.49 (1.47 7.65)	3.49 (1.47 7.65)	3.73 (1.57 8.19)
All except leukemia[a]	1.67 (1.46 1.92)	1.72 (1.46 2.03)	1.23 (1.00 1.50)
Esophagus	1.15 (0.34 2.33)	1.12 (0.15 2.74)	0.87 (0.11 2.03)
Stomach	1.45 (1.11 1.89)	1.30 (0.93 1.80)	1.00 (0.68 1.43)
Colon	1.66 (0.75 3.02)	2.39 (1.01 4.85)	
Lung	1.62 (1.09 2.28)	1.57 (0.93 2.40)	1.64 (1.06 2.37)
Bladder and urinary tract	2.83 (1.19 6.02)	4.30 (1.78 11.01)	5.55 (1.17 89.74)
Female breast	4.01 (2.64 6.09)	3.81 (2.42 5.98)	2.52 (0.78 6.22)
Uterus	0.93 (0.57 1.36)	0.75 (0.40 1.15)	0.99 (0.34 1.86)
Rectum	1.94 (0.96 3.39)	1.98 (0.89 3.69)	
Pancreas	3.01 (1.52 5.69)	2.19 (0.68 5.17)	
Liver	1.29 (0.62 2.21)	1.35 (0.64 2.31)	
Gallbladder	0.76 (0.08 1.69)	0.83 (0.09 1.87)	
Ovary	0.48 (0.00 1.47)	1.06 (0.00 3.45)	
Prostate	2.15 (0.91 4.28)	2.26 (0.89 4.74)	
Thyroid	3.23 (2.02 5.03)	3.56 (2.17 5.73)	
Multiple myeloma	3.53 (1.11 9.95)	3.51 (0.64 13.06)	
Other lymphatic tissue	0.77 (0.22 1.50)	0.99 (0.29 1.99)	

[a] 0 rad used instead of 0–9 rad (90% confidence interval).

tality). Regardless of ascertainment method, relative risk was significantly increased for all malignancies, leukemia, all malignancies except leukemia, and cancer of the bladder, urinary tract, and thyroid in Nagasaki. In addition, significantly increased relative risks based on all methods of ascertainment were found for cancer of the stomach, lung, female breast, and pancreas, and multiple myeloma. Generally, estimates of relative risk derived by different ascertainment methods were similar.

As previously reported (*7, 9, 16*), a significant dose-response relationship pattern was observed for leukemia and cancer of the stomach, colon, liver, lung, breast, thyroid, prostate, and urinary tract, and multiple myeloma, as well as for all cancer sites (Fig. 3).

Estimates of absolute risk (excess cases per 10^6 person-year-rad (PYR)) were calculated under the assumption that the risk increases linearly with dose. The estimates based on three different ascertainment sources (all, confirmed, mortality) are shown in Table V. While relative risk estimates showed little differences by source of ascertainment, three estimates of absolute risk varied markedly. For all cancer sites, the absolute risk estimated from all sources was from two to five times higher than the risk estimated from mortality data only. Among various cancer sites, breast cancer showed the largest increase in absolute risk based on all methods over that based on mortality, followed by cancer of the stomach, lung, and uterus. Thus, absolute risk based on mortality data may underestimate the true risks for certain types of cancer. This may occur when cancer incidence is significantly higher than mortality. Such cancer may include relatively low lethal malignancies (such as breast cancer) and those with high incidence (*e.g.*, stomach and lung cancer).

Chronological changes of cancer risk in A-bomb survivors are of special interest for determining how long it takes before clinically evident cancer appears after radiation and

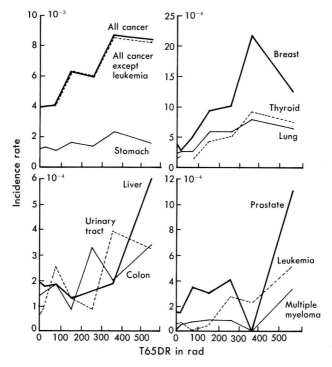

FIG. 3. Nagasaki Tumor Registry. Age-adjusted average annual incidence rate by dose for selected cancer sites, all methods of ascertainment, 1959–78.

TABLE V. Excess Cases per 10^6 PYR for All and Selected Cancer by Method of Ascertainment: Nagasaki, 1959–78

Site	Source					
	All sources		Confirmed		Mortality	
All sites[a]	10.31 (	8.27 12.35)	7.43 (	5.70 9.17)	2.08 (	0.60 3.55)
Leukemia	0.66 (	0.41 0.92)	0.66 (	0.41 0.92)	0.65 (	0.41 0.90)
All except leukemia[a]	9.64 (	7.62 11.67)	6.77 (	5.05 8.48)	1.42 (−0.03	2.87)
Esophagus	−0.07 (−0.38	0.23)	−0.04 (−0.28	0.20)	−0.07 (−0.34	0.19)
Stomach	1.49 (	0.38 2.59)	0.65 (−0.24	1.54)	0.23 (−0.60	1.06)
Colon	0.41 (	0.04 0.77)	0.38 (	0.08 0.69)	0.16 (−0.09	0.40)
Lung	0.87 (	0.27 1.48)	0.65 (	0.16 1.14)	0.55 (	0.01 1.09)
Bladder and urinary tract	0.53 (	0.22 0.84)	0.60 (	0.32 0.88)	0.20 (	0.01 0.40)
Female breast	3.30 (	2.45 4.16)	2.57 (	1.78 3.36)	0.31 (−0.12	0.73)
Uterus	0.09 (−1.01	1.18)	−0.45 (−1.45	0.56)	−0.24 (−0.81	0.33)
Rectum	0.34 (−0.03	0.71)	0.20 (−0.14	0.55)		
Pancreas	0.32 (−0.01	0.66)	0.03 (−0.22	0.28)		
Liver	0.45 (	0.04 0.86)	0.49 (	0.09 0.89)		
Gallbladder	−0.11 (−0.43	0.21)	−0.06 (−0.35	0.24)		
Salivary	−0.06 (−0.19	0.07)	−0.06 (−0.19	0.07)		
Ovary	−0.18 (−0.58	0.21)	−0.14 (−0.52	0.23)		
Thyroid	1.32 (	0.88 1.76)	1.31 (	0.90 1.72)		
Multiple myeloma	0.38 (	0.17 0.60)	0.19 (	0.03 0.34)		
Other lymphatic tissue	0.00 (−0.33	0.33)	0.11 (−0.19	0.40)		

[a] 0 rad used instead of 0–9 rad (90% confidence interval).

TABLE VI.   Excess Incidence/10^6 PYR and 90% Confidence Limits by Period for
Selected Sites of Cancer, Nagasaki, 1959–78

Period	Leukemia	All cancer except leukemia	Stomach
1959–62	2.29 (1.71 2.87)	7.97 (4.60 11.33)	1.83 (−0.04 3.71)
63–66	0.41 (−0.02 0.85)	6.10 (1.85 10.36)	1.26 (−1.12 3.63)
67–70	0.47 (−0.24 1.18)	7.24 (2.72 11.76)	0.42 (−2.29 3.14)
71–74	−0.08 (−0.37 0.22)	9.26 (4.11 14.41)	0.94 (−1.59 3.46)
75–78	−0.37 (−1.10 0.35)	19.65 (14.23 25.08)	2.91 (0.02 5.80)

Period	Lung	Breast	Thyroid
1959–62	1.46 (0.68 2.25)	−0.41 (−1.81 1.00)	2.34 (1.49 3.19)
63–66	0.54 (−0.64 1.72)	0.99 (−0.44 2.43)	1.11 (−0.10 2.32)
67–70	0.82 (−0.66 2.29)	8.62 (6.66 10.58)	0.71 (−0.19 1.61)
71–74	0.77 (−0.85 2.39)	1.95 (−0.27 4.18)	1.33 (0.37 2.30)
75–78	0.79 (−0.87 2.45)	5.86 (3.35 8.38)	1.56 (0.65 2.47)

(90% confidence interval).

how long carcinogenic effects of radiation persist. Table VI presents chronological change in absolute risk of leukemia and several other cancer sites. The excess incidence of leukemia decreased with time and reached zero by 1971, however, the excess risk for malignancies other than leukemia generally increased with time. Various reasons can be considered for the different latency periods for different tumors. For example, for malignancies such as lung and stomach cancer, radiation may play a relatively small role as compared with other initiating and promoting factors (*e.g.*, cigarette smoking, diet, and occupation). Host susceptibility such as age and endocrine factors may also be a significant factor in determining the time of clinical onset of some tumors (*e.g.*, breast and thyroid cancer).

The long-term follow-up of A-bomb survivors offers a unique opportunity for study of the latency period of cancer because of the well-defined time of single exposure. In determining the onset of cancer, incidence data provide a distinct advantage over mortality data. When using mortality data, one must assume that the case fatality or survival rate for a given type of tumor does not differ over calendar time and among different subgroups of interest (*e.g.*, age, sex, *etc.*). Such assumptions are not always justifiable.

Presentation of detailed incidence findings for specific types of cancer is beyond the scope of this paper and are discussed elsewhere in this monograph. However, it seems clear from what is already presented that incidence monitoring must be part of the continuing surveillance of health effects of A-bomb radiation exposure. Incidence data are needed 1) to assess the risk of developing relatively low lethal tumors such as cancer of the breast, thyroid, corpus uteri, *etc.*, 2) to improve diagnostic accuracy for both nonfatal (such as those mentioned above) and fatal (*e.g.*, pancreatic) cancer, and 3) to assess secular changes in carcinogenic effects of radiation. Tissue registry data should provide a unique opportunity for studying histological presentations of radiation-induced tumors, although these data have not been fully utilized. Reasons for difficulty in using tissue registry data include the possible selectivity of cases with histological diagnosis and the lack of clinical and other medical information needed for determining primary sites. The linkage of tumor and tissue registries should help resolve some of the problems.

REFERENCES

1. American Cancer Society. Manual of Tumor Nomenclature and Coding (1968). American Cancer Society, Inc., New York.

2. Belsky, J. L., Takeichi, N., Yamamoto, T., Cihak, R. W., Hirose, F., Ezaki, H., Inoue, S., and Blot, W. J. Salivary gland neoplasms following atomic radiation: Additional cases and reanalysis of combined data in a fixed population, 1957–1970. *Cancer*, **35**, 555–559 (1975).

3. Freedman, L. A., Fukushima, K., and Seigel, D. G. ABCC-JNIH Adult Health Study, Report 4, 1960–62 cycle examination, Hiroshima and Nagasaki. ABCC Tech. Rep. 20-63 (1963).

4. Hanai, A., Kitamura, H., Fukuma, S., and Fujimoto, I. (ed.) Cancer incidence in Japan 1975–1979 (1984). The Osaka Cancer Registry, Osaka.

5. Harada, T., Ide, M., Ishida, M., and Troup, G. M. Malignant Neoplasms, Tumor Registry Data. Hiroshima and Nagasaki 1957–59. Report of the Research Committee on Tumor Statistics, Hiroshima and Nagasaki City Medical Association. ABCC Tech. Rep. 23-63 (1963).

6. Harada, T. and Ishida, M. Neoplasms among A-bomb survivors in Hiroshima; First Report of the Research Committee on Tumor Statistics, Hiroshima City Medical Association, Hiroshima, Japan. *J. Natl. Cancer Inst.*, **25**, 1253–1264 (1960).

7. Ichimaru, M., Ishimaru, T., and Belsky, J. L. Incidence of leukemia in atomic bomb survivors belonging to a fixed cohort in Hiroshima and Nagasaki, 1950–71: Radiation dose, years after exposure, age at exposure, and type of leukemia. *J. Radiat. Res.*, **19**, 262–282 (1978).

8. Ishida, M. Statistical Aspect of Tumor Registries in Hiroshima and Nagasaki. *Bull. Int. Stat. Inst.*, **38**, 233–234 (1961).

9. Kato, H. and Schull, W. J. Studies of the mortality of A-bomb survivors. Report 7. Mortality 1950–1978: Part I. Cancer mortality. *Radiat. Res.*, **90**, 395–432 (1982).

10. Kerr, G. D. and Soloman, D. L. The epicenter of the Nagasaki weapon: A reanalysis of available data with recommended values. Oak Ridge National Laboratory, Oak Ridge, TN, 1976.

11. Maclennan, R., Muir, C. S., Steinitz, R., and Winkler, A. (ed.) Cancer Registration and Its Techniques. International Agency for Research on Cancer (IARC) Scientific Publication No. 21 (1978).

12. Matsuura, H., Yamamoto, T., Sekine, I., Ichi, Y., and Otake, M. Pathological and epidemiological study of gastric cancer in atomic bomb survivors, Hiroshima and Nagasaki, 1955–57. *Radiat. Res.*, **25**, 111–129 (1984).

13. McGregor, D. H., Land, C. E., Choi, K., Tokuoka, S., Lin, P. I., Wakabayashi, T., and Beebe, G. W. Breast cancer incidence among atomic bomb survivors, Hiroshima and Nagasaki, 1950–69. *J. Natl. Cancer Inst.*, **59**, 799–811 (1977).

14. Nakatsuka, H. and Ezaki, H. Colorectal cancer among atomic bomb survivors, this volume, pp. 157–167.

15. Schull, W. J. and Masaki, K. Dosimetry studies information. Documents prepared for RERF seventh meeting of the scientific councillors, 17–19 March 1980.

16. Tokunaga, M., Norman, J. E., Jr., Asano, M., Tokuoka, S., Ezaki, H., Nishimori, I., and Tsuji, Y. Malignant breast tumors among atomic bomb survivors, Hiroshima and Nagasaki, 1950–74. *J. Natl. Cancer Inst.*, **62**, 1347–1359 (1979).

17. Wakabayashi, T., Kato, H., Ikeda, T., and Schull, W. J. Studies of the mortality of A-bomb survivors, Report 7. Part III. Increase of cancer in 1959-1978, based on the Tumor Registry, Nagasaki. *Radiat. Res.*, **93**, 112–146 (1983).

18. Wanebo, C. K., Johnson, K. G., Sato, K., and Thorslund, T. W. Breast cancer after ex-

posure to the atomic bombings of Hiroshima and Nagasaki. *N. Engl. J. Med.*, **279**, 667–671 (1968).

19. Wanebo, C. K., Johnson, K. G., Sato, K., and Thorslund, T. W. Lung cancer following atomic radiation. *Am. Rev. Respir. Dis.*, **88**, 778–787 (1968).
20. World Health Organization. International Classification of Diseases for Oncology (1976). WHO, Geneva.
21. World Health Organization. Manual of the International Statistical Classification of Diseases. Injuries and Causes of Death (1977). WHO, Geneva.
22. Wood, J. W., Tamagaki, H., Neriishi, S., Sato, T., Sheldon, W. F., Archer, P. G., Hamilton, H. B., and Johnson, K. G. Thyroid carcinoma in atomic bomb survivors, Hiroshima and Nagasaki. *Am. J. Epidemiol.*, **89**, 4–14 (1969).
23. Yamamoto, T., Nishimori, I., Tahara, E., and Sekine, I. Malignant tumors in atomic bomb survivors with special reference to the pathology of stomach and lung cancer, this volume, pp. 145–156.

GANN Monograph on Cancer Research 32, 1986

THE CANCER REGISTRY IN NAGASAKI CITY, WITH ATOMIC BOMB SURVIVOR DATA, 1973–1977

Takayoshi Ikeda, Ichiro Hayashi, Takeshi Matsuo,
Hiroshi Maeda, and Isao Shimokawa

*First Department of Pathology, Nagasaki University School of Medicine**

The tumor registry program in Nagasaki City was conceived as a contribution to knowledge concerning possible radiation induced carcinogenesis among a human population and a tumor registry was established in 1957 and a tissue registry in 1974.

According to the chronological changes in adjusted incidence rates for Nagasaki City, an increasing trend was shown in males for cancer of the colon, rectum, lung, urinary bladder, and for all sites combined, and, in females for cancer of the colon, pancreas, and breast. No decreasing trend was observed for any site in males, while a decreasing trend was indicated in females for cancer of the uterus.

In comparison with age-adjusted incidence rates for all cancer sites combined in other prefectures and cities in 1979, the rates in Nagasaki City are high for both males and females. Sites with a tendency for high rates, in Nagasaki City, are, for males, stomach, colon, rectum, liver, and lymphoid tissue, and for females, colon, rectum, liver, gallbladder, lung, breast, and lymphoid tissue.

From these data, it is necessary to ascertain whether or not the incidence of malignant tumors is higher among atomic bomb (A-bomb) survivors than in nonexposed persons. According to the Nagasaki City tumor and tissue registry data for 1973–77, the crude incidence rate and relative risk for several cancers were higher in A-bomb survivors and well correlated with the radiation dose. However, the adjusted relative risk showed a higher trend only for thyroid cancer in females and in double cancers for both sexes. Histopathological difference between cancer tissue of A-bomb survivors and nonexposed persons was not detected.

In general, it is premature to determine the qualitative and quantitative differences of malignancy between A-bomb survivors and nonexposed persons, although an increase in cancer incidence and mortality is a recognized late effect of exposure to A-bomb radiation in Hiroshima and Nagasaki.

The purpose of a population based cancer registry is to determine the magnitude of the effect of tumors, especially malignant tumors, on the community so as to help control the malignancy. Registration is an effective means of epidemiological research to inquire into the cause of malignant tumors, and provides data concerning geopathological differences in carcinogenesis in establishing an epidemiological hypothesis.

The specific purpose of the Nagasaki City Tumor Registry is to ascertain whether or

---

* Sakamoto-machi 12-4, Nagasaki 852, Japan (池田高良, 林 一郎, 松尾 武, 前田 公, 下川 功).

not the incidence of malignant tumors is higher among atomic bomb (A-bomb) survivors than in nonexposed populations.

The Nagasaki City Tumor Statistics Committee was established in Nagasaki City in 1957 as a special committee of the Nagasaki City Medical Association, and tumor registration has been conducted in cooperation with the Radiation Effects Research Foundation (RERF, formerly the Atomic Bomb Casualty Commission) for 27 years. In September 1974, the Nagasaki Neoplasm Tissue Registry Commission was established with a research grant from the U.S. National Cancer Institute, and tissue registration has been carried out jointly.

To improve the accuracy of tumor registration, the use of the International Classification of Diseases (ICD-O) code was recommended in 1976 and a tendency has developed to use this code throughout the world. Histological type has to be considered in epidemiological and clinical studies because it is often related to etiology and prognosis and the ICD-O code makes histological typing of all malignant tumors possible. However, because ICD-O is a classification of histological type, participation of at least one pathologist is necessary in its use. For example, terminology and diagnostic criteria often differ among schools and ICD evaluation by pathologists is necessary. In Nagasaki City, the tissue registry was established in addition to the tumor registry, and these two committees are cooperating.

Population Based Cancer Registry Data

Population based cancer registration is conducted in 13 prefectures and 2 cities in Japan (*2, 8, 9*). One of the main purposes of a population based cancer registration is

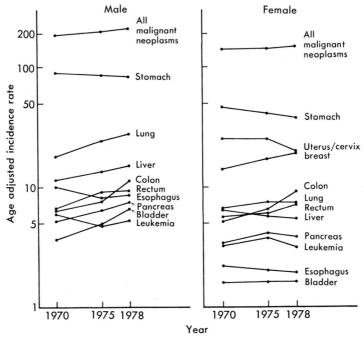

FIG. 1. Chronological changes in estimated incidence rate, Japan 1970, 1975, and 1978.

to determine incidence rates and observe chronological changes. Cancer registration establishes the direction of cancer countermeasures and contributes to epidemiological research on cancer. In Japan, few registry offices possess long period incidence data with moderate accuracy. In these 13 prefectures and 2 cities, both incidence and mortality rates show a slight but gradual rising tendency in recent years as shown in Fig. 1 (2). According to the chronological changes in age-adjusted incidence rates for main cancer sites in Nagasaki, an increasing trend is shown in males for the colon, rectum, lung, urinary bladder, and all sites combined, and an increasing trend in females for the colon, pancreas, and breast. No decreasing trend is observed for any site in males, while a decreasing trend is indicated in females for cancer of the uterus. A peculiar finding in Nagasaki is no decreasing trend for stomach cancer in males compared with other regions.

The proportion of cases based only on death certificates is used as an index of the

TABLE I.   Chronological Changes of the Rate of Cases Based on the Death Certificate
in Four Regions of Japan (% of Cases with Malignancy)

Region	Year					
	1975	1976	1977	1978	1979	1980
A	23.9	21.5	21.8	18.3	16.5	14.1
B	29.2	26.5	29.0	28.5	26.0	26.6
C	22.9	19.6	21.5	15.3	14.1	14.5
D[a]	10.4	8.2	8.0	3.0	9.0	6.1

[a] Nagasaki City.

TABLE II.   Chronological Changes of the Rate of Cases Based on Histological Diagnosis
in Four Regions of Japan (% of All Malignancies)

Region	Year					
	1975	1976	1977	1978	1979	1980
A	58.0	59.6	59.1	64.2	64.1	69.1
B	38.5	43.1	43.0	51.2	56.7	58.4
C	69.4	69.4	63.6	69.3	69.4	72.4
D[a]	67.1	67.1	72.9	76.2	74.3	77.0

[a] Nagasaki City.

TABLE III.   Incidence and Mortality Rates for All Sites by Sex in Six Regions of Japan, 1979

Region	Male		Female	
	Incidence	Mortality	Incidence	Mortality
A	218.7	148.8	142.9	85.2
E	218.5	156.6	140.1	90.2*
F	183.0	145.5	122.8**	84.5
B	220.2	160.5*	148.0	91.6*
C	310.8*	153.7	219.5*	80.2
D	266.2*	177.2*	174.2*	100.6*
Mean	207.1	150.4	141.2	86.7
S.D.	11.7	3.7	8.2	1.7

* mean+2 S.D.
** mean−2 S.D.

T. IKEDA ET AL.

TABLE IV. Adjusted Incidence Rates by Sex and Site[a] in Four Regions of Japan, 1979

ICD	Site	Male				Female			
		A	B	C	D[b]	A	B	C	D[b]
140–209	All malignant neoplasms	218.7	220.2	310.8	266.2	142.9	148.0	219.5	174.2
150	Esophagus	13.6	7.9	11.6	9.2	3.7	1.9	1.9	1.1
151	Stomach	82.0	73.9	98.9	88.9	35.9	37.8	43.6	37.1
153	Colon	8.0	9.8	14.0	13.4	8.9	7.2	10.7	10.6
154	Rectum	9.4	9.4	16.3	10.9	7.2	5.4	9.2	10.0
155	Liver	11.6	25.9	20.9	27.1	4.3	7.0	8.7	11.1
156	Gallbladder, bile duct	6.6	3.7	3.5	7.4	5.6	3.8	3.2	7.3
157	Pancreas	10.6	7.1	8.8	5.4	5.4	4.8	4.3	3.1
161	Larynx	1.7	4.0	7.3	3.1	0.2	0.5	0.7	0.3
162	Lung	30.3	32.8	43.0	30.2	8.3	10.5	12.2	10.7
174, 175	Breast	0.2	0.2	0.0	0.4	21.0	17.3	36.2	22.7
179–182 233.1	Uterus Cervix *in situ* }	—	—	—	—	15.9	27.1	40.3	27.2
183.0	Ovary	—	—	—	—	4.2	3.7	6.3	6.1
185	Prostate	5.7	4.7	9.1	9.4	—	—	—	—
188	Bladder	6.5	6.0	12.1	15.4	1.6	1.8	3.1	2.2
200–203	Lymphatic except leukemia	6.6	5.1	11.4	9.3	4.0	3.6	4.9	6.6
204–208	Leukemia	6.1	4.7	8.2	5.5	3.8	3.2	3.4	0.0
233.1	Cervix *in situ*	—	—	—	—	2.4	4.3	5.9	2.2

[a] Adjusted to world population.
[b] Nagasaki City.

TABLE V. Adjusted Mortality Rates by Sex and Site[a] in Four Regions of Japan, 1979

ICD	Site	Male				Female			
		A	B	C	D[b]	A	B	C	D[b]
140–209	All malignant neoplasms	148.8	160.5	153.7	177.2	85.2	91.6	80.2	100.6
150	Esophagus	10.6	6.4	4.5	4.5	2.5	1.4	1.3	0.0
151	Stomach	48.1	52.5	48.1	43.8	24.3	26.9	24.6	22.6
153	Colon	5.4	6.2	4.9	6.1	4.2	4.7	2.9	4.5
154	Rectum	6.9	6.8	4.5	7.3	5.2	3.6	3.3	5.1
155	Liver	10.4	22.3	21.9	30.1	4.4	6.5	6.4	10.5
156	Gallbladder, bile duct	4.9	3.2	3.3	7.0	5.3	2.9	2.7	6.1
157	Pancreas	9.0	6.2	5.6	6.8	4.3	4.5	3.0	3.4
161	Larynx	1.3	1.6	1.4	0.5	0.4	0.2	0.3	0.0
162	Lung	22.2	28.8	29.1	32.9	7.4	8.8	6.3	9.9
174, 175	Breast	0.1	0.1	0.6	0.0	5.0	5.2	4.9	7.4
179–182 233.1	Uterus Cervix *in situ* }	—	—	—	—	5.3	9.6	8.8	8.9
183.0	Ovary	—	—	—	—	1.9	2.6	3.5	2.9
185	Prostate	2.5	2.3	2.0	2.5	—	—	—	—
188	Bladder	2.5	2.5	2.9	3.2	1.1	0.9	0.7	1.7
200–203	Lymphatic except leukemia	5.2	4.2	5.9	9.9	2.1	2.5	0.9	6.1
204–208	Leukemia	5.2	3.8	5.5	5.7	3.6	2.7	2.5	1.5
233.1	Cervix *in situ*	—	—	—	—	0.0	0.0	0.0	0.0

[a] Adjusted to world population.
[b] Nagasaki City.

accuracy of registration, especially the accuracy of reporting. The reliability of incidence rates is higher when the proportion based only on death certificates is lower. Another index of registration accuracy is the rate of histological diagnosis. The higher the rate of histological diagnosis, the higher becomes the accuracy of the registration. In Nagasaki City, both the proportion of cases based only on death certificates (less than 10%) and the histological diagnosis rate (more than 70%) recently show excellent values (Tables I and II). In comparison with the adjusted incidence rates for all sites among the prefectures and cities in 1979 that are conducting population based cancer registries, the rate is remarkably high in both males and females of Nagasaki City (Table III). The sites showing an increasing tendency of rate in males of Nagasaki City are the stomach, colon, rectum, liver, and lymphoid tissues, and in females, the colon, rectum, liver, gallbladder, lung, breast, and lymphoid tissues (Table IV). Adjusted mortality rates by site (Table V) show a similar trend to adjusted incidence rates (2).

Nagasaki City A-bomb Survivor Data

In general, a higher trend of cancer incidence rates in a certain region is reflected by geographically specific phenomena or by the influence of known or unknown factors, such as air pollution, radiation, *etc.* Geographically, Nagasaki City is located in southwestern Japan by the sea, and a possible factor influencing cancer incidence may be the existence of a particular group (*i.e.*, A-bomb survivors) in the population. The former factor has not been investigated so far, but it has been noted that the frequency of malignant lymphoma, especially the T-cell type, and of liver cancer are higher in Nagasaki Prefecture and in the southwestern part of Japan than in other areas. The pathogenesis of these malignant tumors has been postulated as involvement of viruses, retrovirus or hepatitis B virus. The latter factors have been studied extensively. According to a report on a fixed population of the RERF Life Span Study (LSS) using the tumor registry data in Nagasaki City during the period 1959–78, a higher trend of cancer incidence was noted in several sites, such as leukemia, and cancer of the lung, breast, stomach, and thyroid gland (13). Furthermore, a suggestively higher trend in incidence was observed in cancer of the colon and urinary tract, and in multiple myeloma. In this study, the dose estimates were based on the RERF revised T65 dose system.

As previously described, the rate of histological diagnosis in Nagasaki City was more than 70% for all sites combined in recent years and it may be enough to evaluate the histological types of malignancy in the population by exposure status. For this reason, the authors have investigated, in addition to the population based incidence rates, the pathohistological type of malignancy in several organs by exposure status of survivors in Nagasaki City for five years (1973–77). An exposed person was defined as one who was exposed to the A-bomb directly within 10,000 m from ground zero or who entered the city within two weeks after the bombing. Data of exposure status was prepared by the Data Center of the A-Bomb Disaster, Nagasaki University School of Medicine. In 1975, the middle year of the investigation period, A-bomb survivors in Nagasaki City numbered about 82,000 (18%) among the population of about 450,000 and most A-bomb survivors were already 30 or more years old. Thus, among the population aged 30 years or more, 37.8% were A-bomb survivors (Table VI). This means A-bomb survivors were reaching or had already reached the so-called "cancer age."

The other problem noted was the age distribution of A-bomb survivors, which was

TABLE VI. Population of Nagasaki City, 1975

	Population	Male	Female	Total	Sex ratio
A	Total	214,005	236,189	450,194	0.91
B	Age 30 years or more	99,049	117,746	216,795	0.84
C	A-bomb survivors	33,037	48,964	82,001	0.67
D	C/B (%)	33.4	41.6	37.8	—

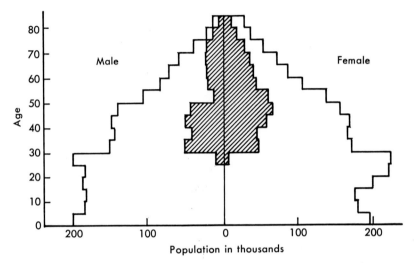

FIG. 2. Age distribution of Nagasaki city population, 1975. ▨, exposed; ☐, non-exposed.

TABLE VII. Incidence of Malignancy and Rates for Histological Diagnosis in Cases Aged 30 Years or More with Malignancy by Exposure Status, Nagasaki City, 1973–77

Sex	Site	Number of cases			Histological diagnosis rate	
		Exposed	Nonexposed	Total	Exposed	Nonexposed
Male	Stomach	302	592	894	78.8	68.8
	Lung	110	196	306	71.8	70.4
	Thyroid	7	10	17	85.7	100.0
	Colon	34	81	115	79.4	61.7
	Multiple	18	25	43	71.7	
Female	Stomach	219	311	530	73.5	65.3
	Lung	60	69	129	66.7	55.1
	Thyroid	31	41	72	96.8	90.2
	Colon	50	58	108	68.0	58.6
	Multiple	25	26	51	76.2	

not regular compared with that of the nonexposed people (Fig. 2). In 1975 a peculiar difference was the decrease of males aged 50–65, and the proportion of people aged more than 75 years was high in the exposed group. It is important to note, for this reason, that the data obtained must be carefully adjusted by age. Possible bias other than age would be the accuracy of tumor registration, especially the rate of histological diagnosis and of the diagnosis only by death certificates. The rate of histological diagnosis was somewhat different between the exposed and nonexposed (Table VII). A-bomb survivors had received more histological examinations for most sites affected, but the difference from the nonexposed was not significant. The incidence and the rate of histological diagnosis of malignant tumors of the stomach, lung, thyroid, and colon, and multiple primary malignant tumors are shown in Table VII. Multiple primary malignancy was regarded as the second or third malignancy detected during the period 1973–77. Histological diagnosis was obtained from tissue registry data in most cases, and some were from observation of microscopic preparations.

1. Stomach cancer (4)

There were 1,424 cases (521 exposed and 903 nonexposed) of stomach cancer registered during the five-year period (Tables VIII and IX). The incidence of stomach cancer tended to be higher in A-bomb survivors exposed within 2,000 m from ground zero, especially in young people, than in the nonexposed but not significantly different. The relative risk was 1.72 for A-bomb survivors and showed a dose-dependent relationship. Age-adjusted relative risk for A-bomb survivors exposed within 2,000 m was 1.28 in males and 1.11 in females, but no difference was noted in the distally exposed or early entrants. Furthermore, the number of cases by age group and histological type was sufficient to permit more detailed study. Relative risk by age for survivors showed higher values in younger people. Incidence by histological type according to Lauren's classification and location for stomach cancer showed no significant difference statistically between A-bomb survivors and nonexposed individuals.

TABLE VIII. Incidence Rates and Relative Risk (vs. nonexposed) for Stomach Cancer in Cases Aged 30 Years or More by Exposure Status and Sex, Nagasaki City, 1973–77

Sex	Rate and risk	Exposure (distance from ground zero)				Nonexposed
		<2,000 m	2,000–9,999 m	Early entry	Total	
Male	Crude incidence rate[a]	277.0	168.1	224.3	191.2	111.3
	Relative risk	2.49	1.51	2.02	1.72	1.00
	Age-adjusted relative risk	1.28	0.84	0.80	0.89	1.00
Female	Crude incidence rate[a]	120.7	86.5	108.4	93.1	54.1
	Relative risk	2.23	1.60	2.01	1.72	1.00
	Age-adjusted relative risk	1.11	0.79	0.84	0.87	1.00

[a] Incidence rate per 100,000.

TABLE IX. Relative Risk (vs. nonexposed) for Stomach Cancer by Exposure Status, Age, and Sex, Nagasaki City, 1973–77

Sex	Exposure (distance from ground zero)	Age in years							
		30–39	40–49	50–59	60–69	70–79	80+	<50	50+
Male	<2,000 m	2.01	1.80	1.56	1.19	1.11	1.37	3.37	1.64
	2,000–9,999 m	0.44	0.84	0.89	0.88	0.91	1.06	1.15	1.33
	Early entry		1.00	0.93	0.75	0.81	0.55	1.84	1.06
	Total	0.54	1.00	0.98	0.88	0.91	0.98	1.49	1.29
Female	<2,000 m	6.73	1.96	0.89	1.66	0.50		4.50	1.01
	2,000–9,999 m	2.18	0.99	0.62	0.83	0.63	1.13	1.85	0.82
	Early entry		0.58	1.06	1.31	0.43	1.81	0.87	1.00
	Total	2.37	1.09	0.72	0.99	0.59	1.10	2.06	0.86

2. *Lung cancer (3)*

There were 435 cases (170 exposed and 265 nonexposed) of lung cancer registered (Table X). Crude incidence rate was higher in A-bomb survivors for both sexes, but no significant difference in the age-adjusted rate was noted compared with nonexposed persons. Relative risk was slightly higher in the exposed, especially for early entrants of both sexes, although age-adjusted relative risk was not significant. The incidence rate by age group was not significant between the exposed and nonexposed. By histological type, adenocarcinoma was the most frequent in both sexes and in both the exposed and nonexposed, followed by squamous cell carcinoma, large cell carcinoma including mucin-like contents, and small cell carcinoma. In A-bomb survivors, adenocarcinoma was more frequent in males and less frequent in females compared with the nonexposed.

TABLE X. Incidence Rates, Relative Risk, and Age-adjusted Relative Risk (*vs.* nonexposed) for Lung Cancer in Cases Aged 30 Years or More, Nagasaki City, 1973–77

Sex	Rate and risk	Exposure (distance from ground zero)					Nonexposed
		<2,000 m	2,000–9,999 m	<9,999 m	Early entry	Total	
Male	Crude incidence rate[a]	66.5	63.7	64.1	104.1	71.6	57.1
	Relative risk	1.17	1.12	1.12	1.83	1.26	1.00
	Age-adjusted relative risk			0.77		0.80	1.00
Female	Crude incidence rate[a]	24.6	25.1	25.1	31.5	26.0	19.3
	Relative risk	1.27	1.30	1.30	1.63	1.35	1.00
	Age-adjusted relative risk			0.90		0.93	1.00

[a] Incidence rate per 100,000.

3. *Thyroid cancer (5)*

There were 89 cases (38 exposed and 51 nonexposed) of thyroid cancer registered (Table XI). The incidence rate tended to be higher in A-bomb survivors, especially in females, than in the nonexposed. Compared with the nonexposed, the relative risk of incidence was increased in the proximally and distally exposed, but not for early entrants. Among 83 cases examined histologically, papillary adenocarcinoma was predominant, and was more prevalent in the exposed than in the nonexposed. Age distribution of the exposed was similar to the nonexposed.

TABLE XI. Incidence Rates and Relative Risk (*vs.* nonexposed) for Thyroid Cancer in Cases Aged 30 Years or More by Exposure Status and Sex, Nagasaki City, 1973–77

Sex	Rate and risk	Exposure (distance from ground zero)			Nonexposed
		<2,000 m	2,000–9,999 m	Early entry	
Male	Crude incidence rate[a]	5.5	4.7	3.5	2.9
	Relative risk	1.90	1.60	1.19	1.00
Female	Crude incidence rate[a]	24.6	12.0	9.5	8.9
	Relative risk	2.75	1.34	1.06	1.00

[a] Incidence rate per 100,000.

4. *Colon cancer (11)*

There were 223 cases (84 exposed and 139 nonexposed) of colon cancer registered.

The incidence in A-bomb survivors was not significantly different compared with the nonexposed. By site, cancer of the sigmoid colon was more frequent in males than in females, particularly in the older age groups, but no difference was noted by exposure status. The relative risk was 0.96 in males and 1.33 in females, although no significant difference was noted in age-adjusted relative risk. Histologically about 90% of the cases were of relatively differentiated adenocarcinoma, and showed no difference by age, sex, or exposure status.

5. Multiple primary malignancies (7)

There were 94 cases (43 exposed and 51 nonexposed) of multiple primary malignancies registered as the second or third malignancy during 1973–77 (Tables XII and XIII). The rate of histological diagnosis by site was difficult to determine, so the rate for all sites combined was used in this study. The average age at the time of the first and second malignancies was younger in females than in males, and by exposure status, the age at the first and second malignancies was older in male and younger in female A-bomb survivors than in the nonexposed. As far as only double cancers are concerned, the average interval between the occurrence of the first and second malignancies was 0.7 years for exposed males and 3.0 years for exposed females, whereas it was 1.7 years for nonexposed males and 2.7 years for nonexposed females. Thus, more than half of the cases had developed the second tumor within a one year period. Stomach cancer was the most frequent (50%) followed by breast cancer (15%). The incidence rate and relative risk were higher in both sexes of the exposed compared with the nonexposed, and the age adjusted relative risk was 1.27 in males and 1.13 in females.

In summary of the data of A-bomb survivors for 1973–77 (Table XIV), several trends may be suggested or demonstrated as follows: 1) Crude incidence rates and

TABLE XII. Average Age at the Time of First, Second, and Third Malignant Tumor by Exposure Status and Sex, Nagasaki City, 1973–77

Malignant Tumor	Exposed		Nonexposed	
	Male	Female	Male	Female
First	67.2	55.3	62.8	60.0
Second	68.7	58.6	64.6	63.4
Third	64.0	33.0	67.3	66.7

TABLE XIII. Incidence Rates and Relative Risk of Multiple Primary Malignant Tumors in Cases Aged 30 Years or More by Exposure Status and Sex, Nagasaki City, 1973–77

Sex	Rate and risk	Exposure (distance from ground zero)			Nonexposed	Total
		<9,999 m	Early entry	Total		
Male	Crude incidence rate[a]	16.76	14.52	16.35	10.20	12.09
	Relative risk	1.64	1.42	1.60	1.00	1.19
	Age-adjusted relative risk	—	—	1.27	1.00	—
Female	Crude incidence rate[a]	13.16	20.19	14.19	9.53	11.36
	Relative risk	1.38	2.17	1.49	1.00	1.19
	Age-adjusted relative risk	—	—	1.13	1.00	—

[a] Incidence rate per 100,000.

TABLE XIV.   Crude Incidence Rates and Relative Risk by Site and Exposure Status, Cases
Aged 30 Years or More, Nagasaki City, 1973–77

Sex	Site	Incidence			Relative risk	
		Exposed	Nonexposed	X	Not adjusted	Adjusted[a]
Male	Stomach	196.6	171.7	NS	1.72	0.89
	Lung	71.6	57.1	NS	1.26	0.80
	Thyroid	4.6	2.9	NS	1.59	
	Colon	22.1	23.1	NS	0.96	0.68
	Double Cancer	11.7	7.3	NS	1.60	1.27
Female	Stomach	94.7	83.9	S	1.72	0.87
	Lung	26.0	19.3	NS	1.35	0.93
	Thyroid	13.4	8.9	NS	1.51	1.29
	Colon	21.6	16.2	NS	1.33	1.04
	Double Cancer	10.8	7.3	NS	1.48	1.13

X, Mantel-Haenszel test.
[a] Calculated by Miettinen method.
S, Significant vs. nonexposed (<2,000 m).
NS, Not significant vs. nonexposed.

relative risk were higher in A-bomb survivors than those in the nonexposed, but the age-adjusted relative risk was not significantly different between them in most malignant tumors investigated. This does not mean that exposure to radiation is not related to cancer induction during the period investigated. 2) The relative risk of these malignancies was well correlated with the radiation dose (distance from ground zero), and the risk for the early entrants was higher in most sites than the survivors exposed at 2,000 m or more. 3) For stomach cancer the relative risk was higher in younger people exposed to radiation at less than 2,000 m from ground zero. Thus, those exposed to radiation at a younger age might be susceptible to malignancies, although malignancies of other sites were not assessable because of the small number of subjects in each age group examined. 4) In A-bomb survivors, the age adjusted relative risk was higher in females for lung, colon, and thyroid cancer and was higher in males for multiple cancer. 5) For double cancer, the age at the first tumor was higher in exposed males than in nonexposed males, while it was lower in exposed females than in nonexposed females. A similar trend was observed for the second malignancy. The trend of lower age in exposed females might be reflected by the earlier occurrence of inherent cancer in younger females such as cancer of the breast and uterine cervix, but the reason for early or late occurrence of the first and second tumors in females or males of the exposed was not elucidated in this study.

At present, an increase in cancer incidence and mortality is an indisputable late effect of exposure to A-bomb radiation in Hiroshima and Nagasaki. According to a cohort study by RERF, it is demonstrated that mortality from malignant tumors among A-bomb survivors is higher in Hiroshima than in Nagasaki. Furthermore, organs involved in elevated risk of cancer are more numerous in Hiroshima than in Nagasaki (6). These data may indicate that biological effect of exposure to neutrons is generally greater than gamma radiation (1), but the new dosimetry indicates that this interpretation is incorrect.

The histological type of cancer has been suggested to differ in incidence by cause such as environmental factors and sex. The difference in histology between radiation induced cancer and spontaneous cancer is still equivocal at present. For breast cancer, the histological type is not different between the exposed and nonexposed, although the incidence is higher in A-bomb survivors (*12*). A similar situation is observed in stomach cancer where poorly differentiated adenocarcinoma is more frequent in A-bomb survivors than in the nonexposed (*10*). Adenocarcinoma of the lung is more frequent especially in exposed males than in the others (*3*). However, these data are not adequate to be decisive.

Thus, in general, it is premature to determine the qualitative differences of malignancy between A-bomb survivors and the nonexposed. Further investigation and accumulation of data are required.

CONCLUSION

A population based cancer registration is a useful means for detection of the cause or related factors of carcinogenesis. In fact, a cohort study or population based cancer registration has contributed to clarifying a higher trend of malignant lymphoma and liver cancer, and also of malignancy in A-bomb survivors in Nagasaki City. At present, A-bomb survivors are reaching or have reached those ages at which the incidence of cancer is elevated. Under these circumstances, it is necessary to investigate continuously the chronological changes of cancer incidence and the trend of incidence by histological type of malignancy in every organ to evaluate radiation induced carcinogenesis.

Acknowledgments

The authors express their sincere appreciation to all members of the Nagasaki Tumor Registry Committee of the Nagasaki City Medical Association for allowing the use of the registry data on tumors, and to all members of the Department of Epidemiology and Statistics, RERF for providing the cancer registry data. The authors also express their gratitude to Mrs. Mariko Mine, the Data Center for A-Bomb Disaster, Nagasaki University School of Medicine, for providing the data of exposure status.

REFERENCES

1. Fujita, S., Shimizu, Y., Yoshimoto, K., Yoshimoto, Y., and Kato, H. RBE of neutron in cancer mortality among atomic bomb survivors, Hiroshima and Nagasaki, 1950–1978. RERF Tech. Rep. 9-80, 1–19 (1983).
2. Fukuma, S. Studies on the Correlation between Environmental Factors and Treatment of Cancers in Cancer Registries. Progress Report Contract No. 56–2, Ministry of Health and Welfare (1983) (in Japanese).
3. Ide, M., Matsuo, T., Shimokawa, I., Mine, H., Maeda, H., and Ikeda, T. Epidemiology of Lung Cancer in Nagasaki—Especially in relation to radiation exposure. *Jpn. J. Cancer Clin.*, **30**, 334–339 (1984) (in Japanese).
4. Iwasaki, K., Kawamoto, K., Shimokawa, I., Matsuo, T., and Ikeda, T. Epidemiological Studies on Gastric Cancer in Nagasaki *Jpn. J. Cancer Clin.*, **30**, 1746–1754 (1984) (in Japanese).
5. Jubashi, T., Matsuo, T., Shimokawa, I., Wago, M., and Ikeda, T. Epidemiological Studies on Thyroid Cancer in Nagasaki City. *Jpn. J. Cancer Clin.*, **30**, 459–465 (1984) (in Japanese).
6. Kurihara, M., Munaka, M., Hayakawa, N., Yamamoto, H., Ueoka, H., and Ohtaki, M. Mortality Statistics among Atomic Bomb Survivors in Hiroshima Prefecture, 1968–1972. *J. Radiat. Res.*, **22**, 456–471 (1981)

7. Murase, K., Shimokawa, I., Hayashida, M., Matsuo, T., and Ideda, T. Epidemiological Studies on Multiple Primary Malignant Tumors in Nagasaki City. *Jpn. J. Cancer Clin.*, **30**, 871–879 (1984) (in Japanese).

8. Research Group for Population-based Cancer Registration in Japan. Cancer Incidence in Japan, 1975—Cancer Registry Statistics, *In* "Cancer Mortality and Morbidity Statistics" (GANN Monograph on Cancer Research No. 26), ed. M. Segi *et al.*, pp. 92–116 (1981). Japan Sci. Soc. Press, Tokyo.

9. Research Group for Population Based Cancer Registration in Japan. Prediction of the Future Incidence of Cancer in Japan. *Jpn. J. Clin. Oncol.*, **12**, 65–72 (1982).

10. Sekine, I., Nishimori, I., Matsuura, H., Yamamoto, T., and Ochi, Y. Pathological and epidemiological studies of gastric cancer in atomic bomb survivors (1950–1977, Hiroshima and Nagasaki). *Annu. Rep. Res. Assoc. Late Effect A-Bomb*, **23**, 105–112 (1982).

11. Shimokawa, I., Matsuo, T., Matsuo, S. and Ikeda, T. Epidemiological Studies of Colon Cancer in Nagasaki City, with special reference to radiation exposure. *Jpn. J. Cancer Clin.*, **30**, 1269–1273 (1984) (in Japanese).

12. Tokunaga, M., Norman, J. E., Jr., Asano, M., Tokuoka, S., Ezaki, H., Nishimori, I., and Tsuji, I. Malignant breast tumors among atomic bomb survivors, Hiroshima and Nagasaki, 1950–1974. *J. Natl. Cancer Inst.*, **62**, 1347–1359 (1979).

13. Wakabayashi, T., Kato, H., Ikeda, T., and Schull, W. J. Studies of the Mortality of A-Bomb Survivors, Report 7: Part III. Incidence of Cancer in 1959–1978, Based on the Tumor Registry, Nagasaki. *Radiat. Res.*, **93**, 112–146 (1983).

CANCER MORTALITY

Hiroo KATO

Department of Epidemiology and Statistics,
Radiation Effects Research Foundation*

The Radiation Effects Research Foundation (RERF) and its predecessor, the Atomic Bomb Casualty Commission (ABCC), have conducted mortality surveillance on a fixed sample, the Life Span Study (LSS), of 82,000 atomic bomb (A-bomb) survivors and 27,000 nonexposed residents of Hiroshima and Nagasaki since 1950. The results of the most recent analysis of the LSS can be summarized as follows:

1. As a late effect of A-bomb radiation, mortality from malignant tumors increased among A-bomb survivors. Besides, the well-known increase of leukemia, cancer of the lung, breast, stomach, colon, and thyroid, and multiple myeloma also increased, but no increase in mortality from cancer of the rectum and uterus has yet been observed.

2. An increase in leukemia mortality among A-bomb survivors began to appear 2–3 years after exposure and reached a peak within 5–6 years. Thereafter, it decreased. For Hiroshima, however, the mortality rate is still slightly higher than the control level, even in the most recent period of observation from 1974–78. The pattern of appearance over time of radiation-induced cancer other than leukemia, however, differs from that of leukemia. In general, radiation-induced solid cancer begins to appear after the age is attained at which the cancer is normally prone to develop (so-called cancer age), and has continued to increase proportionately with the increase in mortality of the control group as it ages.

3. There are factors which modify the effect of radiation, such as age at the time of the bomb (ATB). Sensitivity to radiation, in terms of cancer induction, is higher for persons who were young ATB in general than for those who were older ATB.

4. The number of excess deaths from cancer among A-bomb survivors has been estimated. Results indicate that 50% of the leukemia deaths and 3.5% of the deaths due to all cancer except leukemia that have occurred in the LSS sample during the period 1950–78 are attributable to A-bomb radiation.

5. The relationship between radiation and other carcinogens such as tobacco has been investigated. There seems to be no interaction in a multiplicative way between radiation and smoking in lung cancer induction. Rather, the joint effect seems more consistent with an additive model.

The Atomic Bomb Casualty Commission (ABCC) and the Radiation Effects Research Foundation (RERF) have conducted mortality surveillance on a fixed sample (Life Span Study (LSS)) of 82,000 atomic bomb (A-bomb) survivors and 27,000 nonexposed residents of Hiroshima and Nagasaki since 1950 (*2, 3*). The LSS was designed to identify and

* Hijiyama Park 5-2, Minami-ku, Hiroshima 732, Japan (加藤寛夫).

measure the possible late effects of acute radiation exposure from the A-bombs expressed through mortality overall or by specific disease categories. Its strength is that mortality ascertainment is essentially complete, regardless of a person's address in Japan, due to the periodic check of Koseki records of the LSS sample members. Its weakness is its reliance on the cause of death as stated on the death certificate. Some of the misclassification that can arise is compensated for by collateral use of autopsy information and data from the Hiroshima and Nagasaki Tissue and Tumor Registries (34).

Periodic analyses of the mortality experience of the LSS sample continue; the most recently published account spanned the years 1950–78 (15, 16). The late effects of A-bomb radiation on mortality have been limited, so far, to an excess mortality from malignant neoplasms and not from other causes of death. No shortening of life-span due to causes other than malignant neoplasms was observed. Thus, the results obtained do not support the nonspecific acceleration of aging due to radiation.

With the ongoing accumulation of data, the most recent analysis addresses problems which previous publications were able to treat less well because of a small number of deaths (16). Issues such as the latent period for radiation-related malignancies and the effects of age at the time of the bomb (ATB) as well as attained age (age at death) on radiation carcinogenesis can now be examined.

As a reassessment of A-bomb dosimetry is currently under way, the shape of the dose response curve for gamma rays or the relative biological effectiveness (RBE) of neutrons based on the current A-bomb dosimetry system (tentative 1965 dose(T65D)) may change. Therefore, results of analyses of dose response and RBE based on the interim revised shielding dose estimates will also be introduced in this paper.

Study Sample

The LSS sample consists of persons who were living in either Hiroshima or Nagasaki at the time of the census of A-bomb survivors conducted by the Japanese government in 1950, five years after the bombing. As originally defined, the sample included 1) most persons who were within 2,500 m of ground zero in either city ATB, 2) a sample of persons who were between 2,500 and 10,000 m from ground zero, and 3) a sample of persons who were not in the city (NIC) or beyond 10,000 m ATB. The latter two samples were matched by city, sex, and age to a core group of survivors who were less than 2,000 m from ground zero ATB. The distribution of the total of 120,132 persons in the LSS sample by radiation dose and city is shown in Table I.

It has been observed that mortality in the NIC group is lower than that observed among survivors who were in the city ATB but received little or no radiation dose (the distally exposed group). It is generally believed that these differences in mortality are

TABLE I.   Number of Subjects of the Extended LSS Sample

City	Total	Nonexposed	T65 dose in rad					
			0	1–9	10–99	100–199	200+	Unknown
Hiroshima	82,064	20,168	27,569	15,931	13,692	1,740	1,538	1,426
Nagasaki	38,068	6,349	15,397	7,137	5,470	1,388	1,369	958
Total	120,132	26,517	42,966	23,068	19,162	3,128	2,907	2,384

Source: Kato and Schull (16).

due to factors other than radiation exposure. For this reason the most recent analyses of LSS data have excluded the NIC group.

Ascertainment of Survival Status and Causes of Death

A family registration system (Koseki) was established in Japan about 100 years ago, under which all vital events which affect a family composition such as birth, death, and marriage are registered at the legal address (Honseki) of the family. Therefore, it is possible to ascertain easily and accurately the survival status of a study subject by checking the Koseki (Honseki) regardless of the actual residence of the person. Ascertainment of death is almost 100% complete in the LSS because the Koseki of the study subjects are checked periodically. Upon learning the fact of death and the address of the deceased as a result of the Koseki check, the cause of death is obtained from the vital statistics death schedule kept at the Health Center in which the address of the deceased is recorded. The vital statistics death schedules are prepared from death certificates, and thus the accuracy of the cause of death is a problem. In comparing the death certificate cause of death and that stated in the autopsy protocol, the latter diagnosis is treated as the true cause. Agreements or disagreements between the two sources of information can be examined in the following terms:

Principal autopsy diagnosis	Underlying cause of death		Total
	Disease X	Other than disease X	
Disease X	a Confirmed	b False negative	a+b
Other than disease X	c False positive	d Absence of disease	c+d
Total	a+c	b+d	a+b+c+d

Four possible outcomes are specified, two agreements (a and d) and two disagreements (b and c). The percentage of cases in which the underlying cause is confirmed by autopsy

TABLE II. Accuracy of Cause of Death for Malignant Neoplasms of Specific Sites, Autopsy Cases among the LSS Sample, 1961–75

Cause of death	Death certificate	Autopsy report	Agreement	Confirmation rate	Detection rate
Malignant neoplasms of:					
Buccal cavity and pharynx	19	17	13	68.4%	76.5%
Esophagus	50	53	36	72.0	67.9
Stomach	444	495	374	84.2	75.6
Large intestine	43	54	28	65.1	51.9
Rectum	45	46	32	71.1	69.6
Liver, gallbladder and bile duct	42	169	26	61.9	15.4
Pancreas	56	81	36	64.3	44.4
Trachea, bronchus, lung	192	172	117	60.9	68.0
Breast	40	49	38	95.0	77.6
Uterus	70	83	57	81.4	68.7
Prostate	13	24	5	38.5	20.8
Urinary organs	38	60	30	78.9	50.0
Malignant lymphoma	40	56	31	77.5	55.4
Leukemia	42	40	36	85.7	90.0

Source: Yamamoto et al. (37).

is called a confirmation rate, defined as $100a/(a+c)$. The complement of the confirmation rate, $100c/(a+c)$ is the false positive rate. Similarly, the rate of correspondence between the underlying cause of death and principal autopsy diagnosis is $100a/(a+b)$, termed the detection rate. Its complement, $100b/(a+b)$ is the false negative rate.

Table II shows the accuracy of the cause of death classification on death certificates as revealed by autopsy findings for those individuals who came to autopsy (37). Shown are the confirmation rate and detection rate by major cancer site. Confirmation and detection rates differ according to the cause of death: the rates are high for cancer such as leukemia, breast, and stomach, being over 70%, but the accuracy is poor for cancer such as the pancreas and liver where the confirmation rate is less than 50%. In studying cancer of sites having low accuracy, it is possible to restrict the study to only those that have been histologically confirmed either through autopsy or surgical pathology.

The underlying cause of death is classified according to the International Classification of Diseases (ICD). The cause of death has been coded by the 7th (1950–65), 8th (1968–78), and 9th (from 1979) revisions of the ICD.

Radiation Dose

The A-bombs dropped on Hiroshima (6 August 1945) and Nagasaki (9 August 1945) were of different design and content. A uranium bomb was used in Hiroshima and a plutonium bomb in Nagasaki. Whereas the radiation generated in Nagasaki consisted almost entirely of gamma rays, neutrons also contributed to the total dose received by survivors in Hiroshima; the amount, however, has recently become a matter of controversy and remains unresolved (28, 33). The dose actually received by individuals differs according to their shielding; the shielding configuration and distance were established by interview for all members of the fixed samples. Their gamma ray and neutron kerma (tissue) doses, with consideration of the attenuation from shielding, were calculated in 1965; these dose estimates are referred to as T65D (22). The number of subjects in the sample by exposure dose is shown in Table I. Those exposed received a kerma dose of 27 rad on the average, but 6,000 individuals received a dose of 100 rad or more.

It must be borne in mind that uncertainty continues to surround both the quantity and quality of the radiation released by these two nuclear devices, particularly the Hiroshima bomb. Only one weapon of the Hiroshima type has ever been detonated and thus its yield has had to be reconstructed from tests and reactor experiments on other weapons. Different reconstructions have led to different estimates of the gamma ray and neutron exposure. A recent reassessment suggests that the gamma ray estimates used in the T65D calculations may be too low and the neutron estimates too high, and that the total kerma dose may have been greater than previously supposed (21), although another dosimetry review (18) differs in some of these particulars. This would have the effect of diminishing the slope of the dose-response curve based on total kerma and would make the results seen in the two cities more similar if these reassessments are correct. Given the uncertainties, attention here is restricted to exposure expressed as total kerma from the T65D estimates since this parameter changes least, relatively, for exposures of 10 rad or more when contrasted with the new dose assessments. Unfortunately, the new calculations are still too incomplete to form the basis of a meaningful dose-response analysis based upon individual exposure assessments. There are, for example, as yet no satisfactory estimates of building shielding factors or tissue attenuation of dose, although these estimates may be expected to change (*28*).

Statistical Methods

The statistical methods used here are described in detail elsewhere (*2*). Briefly, the exposed individuals in the sample (excluding the not-in-city and unknown dose groups) were divided into eight dose categories and a contingency table analysis was conducted adjusting for age ATB, sex, city, and period (year of death) using the Mantel-Haenszel method based on person-years at risk. In addition to the usual chi-square test, Cochran's linear trend chi-square test was calculated for the summary contingency table. Relative risks are defined as the ratios of two quotients, namely, the observed to expected deaths in the 100+ (or 200+) rad group and the observed to expected deaths in the 0 rad group where dose is the simple arithmetic sum of the estimated kerma from gamma rays and neutrons. The absolute risk was calculated from a linear regression of the excess deaths (observed / expected deaths) in each dose group in the summary contingency table using the mean for each dose group as the independent variable.

The cumulative death rates for specific cancer sites were calculated by the life table method considering the competing risk of death from other causes (*9*).

1. Cancer mortality by site

It is well known that the incidence rate of leukemia increased among A-bomb survivors. Mortality from malignant tumors other than leukemia also increased after a minimum incubation period of 10–15 years (*i.e.*, since 1955–60). However, this increase in cancer mortality was not observed for all cancer sites.

Mortality in the high dose group (200+ rad) for the period 1950–78 is presented in Fig. 1 by site as a relative risk based on mortality in the 0 rad group (*2*). A significantly elevated relative risk has been observed for leukemia and multiple myeloma, as well as for cancer of the esophagus, stomach, colon, lung, breast, and urinary tract. No elevation

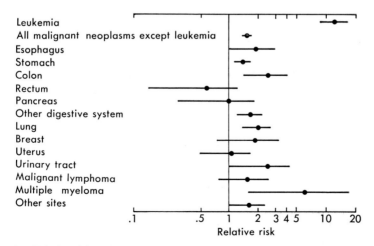

Fig. 1. Relative risk and 90% confidence intervals for specific cancer sites, 1950–78 (200+ rad *vs.* 0 rad).

of risk is evident for cancer of the pancreas, rectum, or uterus, or malignant lymphoma.

Other studies of the same fixed population have shown no increase in chronic lymphatic leukemia (12), liver cancer (1), or intracranial tumors (23). Thus, the sensitivity to radiation differs according to the organ. However, since the risk of cancer, other than leukemia, has increased in the exposed group compared with the controls only after the exposed individuals reach the age at which a cancer is prone to develop (16), and that age differs according to the organ, an increased risk for these cancers may be observed in the future.

In fact, the increase in mortality with dose for cancer of the stomach, esophagus, and urinary tract became significant for the first time with the analysis of mortality from 1950–74 (3). Similarly, the increase in mortality of colon cancer and multiple myeloma became significant only after adding another four years of follow-up and the analysis of mortality from 1950–78 (16). In this regard, the current analysis of mortality through 1982 has revealed for the first time that cancer of the ovary also shows a significant relationship with radiation dose (25). These findings reflect the fact that the number of radiation induced cancers increase with age.

We have used the magnitude of the relative risk of cancer of a particular site as a base, and examined radiation sensitivity by site. As shown in Fig. 1, the 90% confidence limits of the relative risks of breast, stomach, lung, and colon cancer overlap each other and the relative risk of cancer of all sites (except leukemia) is within that confidence limit. This is one indication that the relative risk does not differ according to target organ. However, because the risk may increase in future, careful follow-up will be necessary before any conclusion can be drawn regarding differences in the risk of carcinogenesis by site.

As previously mentioned, the analysis of cancer mortality based on death certificate diagnoses is not adequate for some cancer sites which exhibit a low confirmation rate of diagnosis or a high survival rate. Accordingly, Table III was prepared to classify cancer sites according to the nature of the relationship identified thus far with radiation dose (i.e., an established increase, a suggestive increase, and no increase) (17). In constructing Table III, all sources of material were considered (i.e., mortality, autopsy, and tumor registry data).

Cancer sites which have not yet shown any increase in risk include osteosarcoma and skin cancer. Previously identified increases in risk for these two cancer sites have been

TABLE III.   Relationship with Radiation Dose by Cancer Site

Established increase	Suggestive increase	No increase
Leukemia (except chronic lymphatic)	Cancer of:	Chronic lymphatic leukemia
Cancer of:	Colon	Cancer of:
Thyroid	Esophagus	Bile duct
Breast	Ovary	Gallbladder
Lung	Salivary gland	Intracranium
Stomach	Urinary tract	Liver
Multiple myeloma	Malignant lymphoma	Osteosarcoma
		Prostate
		Skin
		Rectum
		Uterus

Source: Kato and Shigematsu (17).

observed among persons receiving high dose partial-body exposures as part of medical therapy (6). A-bomb survivors, however, received whole-body irradiation of much lower dose.

2. *Latent period of radiation induced cancer*

In general, the time interval between exposure to radiation and the onset of disease is defined as the latent period. In epidemiological studies, however, the exact time of disease onset is often not available. Instead, date of death rather than date of onset is frequently used to determine the latent period. Thus, the period from A-bomb radiation exposure to death from cancer might be regarded as the latent period for radiation-induced cancer, assuming that survival from onset to death is generally uniform between any comparison groups.

It should be noted that it is difficult to determine the latent period in the case of chronic irradiation such as that due to occupational exposure to radiation or exposure to medical X-ray. It is also difficult to follow occupationally exposed subjects for long periods, including after retirement. For these reasons, observation of the A-bomb survivor samples is unique and provides a valuable opportunity to estimate the latent period of radiation induced cancer. For survivors, the time of exposure is known and the ascertainment of mortality is almost complete, as mentioned previously. Radiation induced leukemia began to appear 2–3 years after exposure and reached a peak in 1950–51, decreasing thereafter (12). As shown in Fig. 2, mortality within the high dose group (100+ rad) has decreased since 1950 in both Hiroshima and Nagasaki, reaching the control level during 1971–74 in Nagasaki. For Hiroshima, however, the mortality rate is still higher than that of the control group, even in the latest observation period, 1979–82 (25). Thus, it is roughly estimated that the incubation period of radiation induced leukemia is around 12 years on the average (with a range of 2–35 years).

An example of latent period patterns observed for radiation-induced solid tumors is illustrated in Fig. 3 using lung cancer mortality as a model (16). Shown are the cumulative mortality rates by year, estimated by the life table method and taking into account competing risks, by age ATB for the high dose group (100+ rad) and the 0–9 rad group. The time at which lung cancer mortality increases apparently differs in

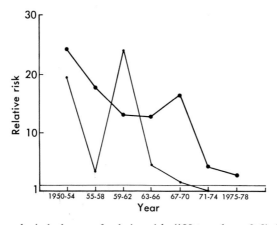

FIG. 2. Chronological change of relative risk (100+ rad *vs.* 0–9) for leukemia deaths by city, 1950–78. ●, Hiroshima; •, Nagasaki.

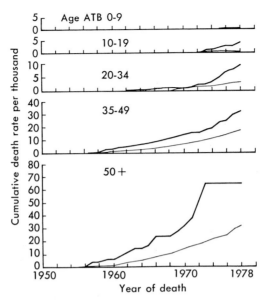

Fig. 3. Cumulative death rate per 1,000 (100+ rad (—) *vs.* 0–9 (—)) for lung cancer by age ATB, 1950–78.

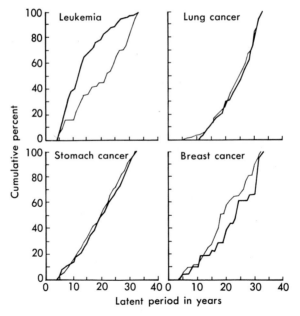

Fig. 4. Cumulative percentage of latent period (100+ rad (—) *vs.* 0 (—)) for specific cancer sites by radiation dose.

the high dose group according to age ATB: radiation-induced lung cancer develops only after the A-bomb survivors attain the age at which this cancer normally develops. This generally occurs at 40 or more years of age, and thus the period from A-bomb exposure to death (latent period) is longer the younger the age ATB. The same tendency is noted with breast and stomach cancer.

posium on Neutron Dosimetry, Gesellschaft für Strahlen-und Umweltforschung, Munich-Neuherberg, June 1–5 (1981).

19. Kurihara, M., Munaka, M., Hayakawa, N., Yamamoto, H., Ueoka, H., and Ohtaki, M. Mortality statistics among atomic bomb survivors in Hiroshima Prefecture, 1968–1972. *J. Radiat. Res.*, **22**, 456–471 (1981).

20. Land, C. E. and Norman, J. E., Jr. Latent periods of radiogenic cancer occurring among Japanese A-bomb survivors. *In* "Late Biological Effects of Ionizing Radiation," Vol. 1, Proceedings of Symposium, Vienna, 13–17 March, IAEA-SM-224/602, pp. 29–47 (1978). International Atomic Energy Agency, Vienna.

21. Loewe, W. E. and Mendelsohn, E. Revised estimates of dose at Hiroshima and Nagasaki, and possible consequences for radiation-induced leukemia. (Preliminary) Report D 80–14 (1980). Lawrence Livermore National Laboratory, California, U.S.A.

22. Milton, R. C. and Shohoji, T. Tentative 1965 radiation dose estimation for atomic bomb survivors, Hiroshima and Nagasaki. ABCC Tech. Rep. 1-68 (1968).

23. Pinkston, J. A., Wakabayashi, T., Yamamoto, T., Asano, M., Harada, Y., Kumagami, H., and Takeuchi, M. Cancer of the head and neck in atomic bomb survivors, Hiroshima and Nagasaki, 1957–76. *Cancer*, **48**, 2172–2178 (1981).

24. Prentice, R. L., Yoshimoto, Y., and Mason, M. W. Relationship of cigarette smoking and radiation exposure to cancer mortality in Hiroshima and Nagasaki. *J. Natl. Cancer Inst.*, **70**, 611–622 (1983).

25. Preston, D. L., Kato, H., Kopecky, K. J., and Fujita, S. Life Span Study, Report 10. Part I. Cancer mortality among atomic bomb survivors, 1950–82. RERF Tech. Rep. 1-86 (1986).

26. Radford, E. P. Statement concerning the current version of cancer risk assessment in the Report of the Advisory Committee on the Biological Effects of Ionizing Radiation (BEIR III committee). BEIR III Report, pp. 287–314 (1980). National Academy Press, Washington, D.C.

27. Rossi, H. H. Separate Statement-Critique of BEIR III. *In* "The Effects on Populations of Exposure to Low Levels of Ionizing Radiation, 1980," pp. 254–260 (1980). National Academy Press, Washington, D.C.

28. Second US-Japan joint workshop for reassessment of atomic bomb radiation dosimetry in Hiroshima and Nagasaki. Proceeding of a workshop held at Hiroshima, 8–9 November 1983 (1983). RERF, Hiroshima.

29. Shore, R. E., Hempelmann, L. H., Kowaluk, E., Mansur, P. S., Pasternack, B. S., Albert, R. E., and Haughie, G. E. Breast neoplasm in women treated with X-ray for acute postpartum mastitis. *J. Natl. Cancer Inst.*, **59**, 813–822 (1977).

30. Stewart, A. and Kneale, G. W. Radiation dose effects in relation to obstetric X-ray and childhood cancers. *Lancet*, **1**, 1185–1188 (1970).

31. Sztanyik, L. B. Late biological effects of A-bombing in Japan. *In* "Late Biological Effects of Ionizing Radiation," Vol. 1, Proceedings of Symposium, Vienna 13–17 March, IAEA-SM-224/602, pp. 61–70 (1978). International Atomic Energy Agency, Vienna.

32. Tokunaga, M., Land, C. E., Yamamoto, T., Asano, M., Tokuoka, S., Ezaki, H., and Nishimori, I. Incidence of female breast cancer among A-bomb survivors, Hiroshima and Nagasaki, 1950–1980. RERF Tech. Rep. 15-84 (1984).

33. US-Japan joint workshop for reassessment of atomic bomb radiation dosimetry in Hiroshima and Nagasaki. Proceeding of a workshop held at Nagasaki, Japan, 16–17 February, ed. Thompson, D. J. (1983). RERF, Hiroshima.

34. Wakabayashi, T., Kato, H., Ikeda, T., and Schull, W. J. Studies of the mortality of A-bomb survivors, Report 7. Part III. Incidence of cancer in 1959–1978, based on the tumor registry, Nagasaki. *Radiat. Res.*, **93**, 112–146 (1983).

35. Watanabe, S. Cancer and leukemia developing among A-bomb survivors. *In* "Handbuch

der allgemeinen pathologie. Geschwülste. Tumors I. Morphologie, Epidemiologie, Immunologie," ed. Grundmann, E., p. 461 (1974). Springer-Verlag, Berlin.

36. Whittemore, A. S. and McMillan, A. Lung cancer mortality among US uranium miners: a reappraisal. *J. Natl. Cancer Inst.*, **71**, 489–499 (1983).

37. Yamamoto, T., Moriyama, I. M., Asano, M., and Guralnick, L. Radiation Effects Research Foundation Pathology Studies, Hiroshima and Nagasaki, Report 4. The Autopsy program and the Life Span Study, January 1961–December 1975. RERF Tech. Rep. 18-78 (1978).

METHODS FOR STUDY OF DELAYED HEALTH EFFECTS OF A-BOMB RADIATION

Edward P. Radford, Dale Preston, and Kenneth J. Kopecky

*Department of Epidemiology and Statistics,
Radiation Effects Research Foundation**

Methods for studying the delayed health effects of ionizing radiation among atomic bomb (A-bomb) survivors have been evolving in recent years. The chief delayed effects of interest are malignant and benign tumors in a defined sample of 93,614 survivors who were in Hiroshima and Nagasaki at the time of the bombing within 10,000 m from ground zero; nearly 65% of this group were in Hiroshima. In addition, a group of children irradiated in utero has been under study. Cancer cases are being identified from the tumor registries in both cities, as well as by death certificate searches; increasing emphasis is being placed on incident cases as well as certain benign tumors, which have been shown to be radiation-related. Previous methods of analysis have generally been by a contingency table technique, in order to compare cancer incidence and mortality rates, and to produce summary measures of risk or descriptions of radiation dose-response relationships. Application of new methods of analysis has been greatly aided by the availability of improved computer resources, as well as development of sophisticated statistical techniques. Examples are the use of hazard rate procedures, with relative and absolute risk models fitted to the data. Potential dose-effect modifiers that can readily be investigated include sex, age at exposure, time since exposure, attained age, and smoking, for example. In addition, a number of case-control studies have been carried out to investigate effects of factors potentially confounding A-bomb radiation effects. In particular, medical radiation exposures have been evaluated.

The follow-up studies of survivors of the atomic bombing in Hiroshima and Nagasaki have now extended for nearly 40 years, the largest prospective human epidemiologic study yet undertaken. In defining the effects of low doses of ionizing radiation, the A-bomb survivor study is especially important because it involves a group of people of all ages and both sexes who were in reasonable health prior to radiation exposure. Moreover, although many people who were near ground zero in both cities received radiation doses well over 100 rad, a high proportion of these did not survive long after the bombing, and therefore the majority of those in the study population of survivors identified in 1950 were exposed to much lower doses. For this reason the average tissue dose for those exposed to 1 rad or more is less than 20 rad, and thus many results are especially relevant to effects of low doses of radiation.

There has been much controversy about interpretation of data from each of the two cities. The two bombs differed in type of nuclear fuel, configuration of the contain-

* Hijiyama Park 5-2, Minami-ku, Hiroshima 732, Japan.

ment, and method of achieving a critical mass at the time of detonation. Until recently it was thought that the type of radiation exposure in the two cities differed significantly, in that the Hiroshima uranium-235 bomb was believed to have a much higher proportion of high energy neutron exposure at ground level than the Nagasaki plutonium-239 bomb. The most recent reassessment of dosimetry (24, 44), however, has indicated that the distribution of high energy neutrons by distance from ground zero was very nearly the same in both cities. Although the free-in-air gamma ray doses continue to be proportionately somewhat higher in Nagasaki compared to Hiroshima at equivalent distances, the neutron component in both cities is now too small to provide any conclusive basis for ascribing differences between results in each city to the quality of radiation exposure. If, as now appears to be the case, there are no significant differences in the radiation effects between the cities with the new doses, then the data for the two cities should be combined with suitable adjustment for differences between the city-specific spontaneous (0 dose) rates. This is advantageous because it increases the precision with which dose-response modification by other factors can be estimated.

This discussion will be restricted to methods appropriate for investigating cancer in the Japanese study populations. Radiation-induced cancer is the principal delayed health effect observed in groups irradiated at whole-body doses well below the acute lethal dose of about 400 rad, and it is also the main focus of this monograph. While the chief emphasis in the studies thus far has been on malignant neoplasms, there is evidence that the risk of certain benign or asymptomatic occult tumors may show an increase with increasing radiation exposure (36). Thus methods of ascertaining benign tumors are important in addition to detection of malignant cancer. Moreover, determination of radiation induction of benign and malignant tumors may throw additional light on the process of human carcinogenesis.

The study of delayed health effects of the bombings in 1945 was developed largely since 1950, and has continued to the present. This period of time has corresponded with a great development of epidemiologic and biostatistical methodology, as techniques of analysis originally developed to investigate epidemics of acute infectious diseases have been improved and extended in their application to chronic diseases such as cancer. Moreover, interest in noninfectious environmental causes of disease has greatly increased, and methods of detecting such environmental factors have become more sophisticated. This evolution of methodologic approaches to study of environmental factors in disease has made available many analytical techniques that were not considered at the time the A-bomb survivor studies were initiated.

Equally important has been the postwar development of extremely versatile and powerful computer technologies, which now permit use of analytical methods well beyond the capability of those available in 1950. The effect of these dramatic developments on the A-bomb studies is to emphasize the importance of reevaluating the analytical methods being applied to the results. Such reevaluation, coupled with the new assessment of radiation dosimetry from the two bombs, has led to important new developments in the study of cancer in the A-bomb survivors, and has altered some of the previously held perceptions concerning risks of radiation-induced cancer.

Study Populations

The primary resource available at Radiation Effects Research Foundation (RERF) for assessment of long-term effects of ionizing radiation is the Life Span Study (LSS) sample; follow-up of this sample began in October 1950. The LSS sample consists of persons who were living in either Hiroshima or Nagasaki at the time of the census of A-bomb survivors conducted by the Japanese government in 1950. As originally defined, the sample included 1) most persons alive at that time who were within 2,500 m from ground zero in either city at the time of the bomb (ATB), 2) a sample of persons who were between 2,500 and 10,000 m from ground zero ATB, and 3) a sample of persons who were not in city (NIC) or beyond 10,000 m. The latter two samples were obtained by matching by sex and age to a group of survivors who were less than 2,000 m from ground zero in each city. The original sample has been extended, most recently in 1982 by the addition of approximately 11,400 distally exposed (2,500–10,000 m) Nagasaki residents for whom complete follow-up data are available. As currently defined, the LSS population contains 120,132 subjects, of whom 38,890 were deceased by the end of 1982. A detailed description of the sample is presented in Beebe and Usagawa (6) and Kato and Schull (23).

An important methodological problem, typical of many epidemiologic studies, has been to define an appropriate control population, with which health effects in those persons exposed to radiation can be compared. In particular, cancer rates have been found in Japan, as elsewhere, to vary considerably by location (15). Thus analyses which compare rates among exposed survivors to national or prefectural cancer rates are of limited value and require careful attention to the possibility of bias. Moreover, it has been observed for many sites that mortality and incidence rates of cancer in the NIC group differ from those observed among survivors who were in the city ATB but received little or no radiation dose from the bombs. These differences in mortality and incidence are thought to arise from factors other than radiation exposure (4). For this reason most recent analyses of the LSS data have excluded the NIC group, and depended on those whose radiation exposure is estimated as zero (or less than 0.5 rad) as the control (non-exposed) population. With the NIC group eliminated, the total study population is presently 93,614 (61,911 in Hiroshima and 31,703 in Nagasaki).

In addition to the LSS population, other groups have been identified for follow-up study in the two cities. Only one of these, a group of 3,643 children who were in utero ATB, is currently considered relevant to the study of radiation-related cancer risks. But another group of potential interest for cancer evaluation is the 76,819 children of men and women who were A-bomb survivors; this group is primarily under study for genetic effects of radiation.

An important subset of the LSS is the Adult Health Study (AHS) population, which has had extensive and continuing clinical evaluations beginning in 1958. This group was selected to include a high proportion of individuals exposed to high doses, and a random sample of survivors with lower doses. In 1958 a total of 19,962 persons were selected from the entire LSS population, as it was then defined. Of these, 16,738 had been examined at least once by the end of 1978 (25). In 1977, another 2,436 persons were added to the AHS population, and over 60% of these were examined at least once within four years (36). All AHS subjects living in or near either city are encouraged to return every two years for detailed evaluation of their health status, including medical history, physical examination, laboratory evaluations, and special clinical studies as needed. The participation rate has declined with successive examination cycles. By the 11th two-year cycle of examinations (July 1978–June 1980) over 30% of the original AHS sample had been lost due to death or migration out of the Hiroshima and Nagasaki contacting areas. However, among the remaining persons, and excluding the NIC group, the participation rate was rather high: the proportion of contactable persons actually examined was 70% in Hiroshima and 85% in Nagasaki (36). For members of the NIC group, who since 1975 have been contacted only by mail, the participation rate had fallen to only 41% in each city by the 11th cycle (36). Altogether 9,387 subjects (7,929 exposed and 1,458 NIC) were examined in that cycle.

Source of Data

The basic data available for each member of the LSS sample are city of residence, sex, and date of birth. For most exposed survivors there are also estimates of the gamma ray and neutron dose received. Those survivors with dose data unassigned numbered 2,386 in 1980, but this number is expected to increase with the adoption of a new dosimetry system. As of this writing the results of radiation dose reevaluations, for which there is fair agreement, indicate the following: 1) As mentioned above, neutron components of the total doses in both cities are so small and so similar that accurate estimation of a differential health effect of gamma rays and neutrons based on intercity comparisons is not feasible. 2) Gamma ray free-in-air doses in Hiroshima are higher by a factor of about 2 to 3 than the old tentative 1965 (T65) doses, while in Nagasaki the free-in-air gamma ray doses are now slightly lower than previously. 3) Shielding by buildings or terrain was much more effective in reducing gamma ray exposure than was thought previously, but shielding by body tissue was somewhat less effective. The net effect is that transmission factors, which are applied to free-in-air gamma ray dose to give tissue dose, are substantially reduced, especially in Nagasaki, where a relatively high percentage of survivors from whom shielding histories were obtained were in factories or shielded by terrain. 4) In comparison with the 1965 dosimetric evaluation (30), the new dosimetry indicates that total radiation doses will be reduced more in Nagasaki than in Hiroshima.

Data on mortality within the LSS sample is obtained by periodic checks of the Japanese system of local family registration offices (Honseki). These offices maintain records of family vital events, births, marriages, deaths, etc., and each living sample member's record (Koseki) is periodically reviewed to determine vital status. Whenever a record of a person's death is found, the date and cause of death are obtained from the vital statistics death schedule at the Health Center for the place of death; the cause of death reported by these centers is obtained from death certificates. Because of the comprehensive nature of the Koseki system, ascertainment of death is believed to be virtually complete for subjects resident in Japan. The hazards of relying on death certificates to establish the primary cause of death are well known. A comparison of certified cause of death and autopsy diagnoses (38, 46) revealed that cancer confirmation and detection rates vary widely according to the type of cancer. The accuracy of death certificates in the LSS population was found to be high for malignant neoplasms of some organs such as breast and stomach, and for leukemia. But for others, such as lung, urinary tract, liver and biliary system, pancreas, and prostate, death certificate data were found to underestimate the presence of cancer considerably (35). This underestimation will produce an equivalent underestimation of the absolute excess risks associated with exposure to radiation. In the AHS sample, ascertainment of cases includes a wide range of disease conditions studied in relation to radiation effects, but in this report we are concerned mainly with benign or malignant tumors.

Data on cancer incidence are also obtained through the tumor registries established in both cities by the local medical societies in the late 1950s, tissue registries in each city, and supplementary case finding efforts conducted for particular studies. At this time reporting of cases by the tumor registries is considered to be good for the two cities. The registries incorporate cases only for those resident in each city at the time of the diagnosis, thus there is underascertainment of cases in the LSS population because of migration out of the cities, a particular problem for those who were young ATB. Data from the AHS population indicate that since 1958 out-migration has been slight (only a few percent). However, prior to that time about 10% of all those living had left. As many as 20% of the members of the youngest age ATB groups may have left the cities prior to 1958. Tokunaga *et al.* (*42*) cited evidence that among AHS females the migration rate was unrelated to radiation dose. Because most of those leaving have settled in the large cities of Honshu and Kyushu, it is possible that they could be traced to tumor registries there, in order to bring the ascertainment of incident cancer closer to 100%.

The cancer incidence data have the advantage that cases are included in the study at the time of diagnosis, often years before fatal cancer would be found from death certificate records. Not only may there be a substantial lag between diagnosis and death, but sometimes as much as two years may elapse before the death certificate data are recorded and detected from the Koseki. The delay in ascertainment from death records is especially important because cancer cases in the LSS are rapidly accumulating, and the evidence of radiation dose-related effects is increasing.

Another important factor in use of tumor registry data is the fact that cases are recorded regardless of outcome. Thus information on nonfatal malignancies and some types of benign tumors can be obtained from the registries. This issue is especially significant for cancer of the thyroid and female breast, which are radiosensitive but not highly fatal. The radiosensitivity of cancer of the prostate is uncertain, in part because ascertainment of cases of cancer of the prostate from death certificates is poor in Japan. Data from the tumor registries, for which ascertainment is somewhat better, indicate a radiation dose-related effect (*43*). Finally, it should be emphasized that use of incident cancer as a basis of defining cancer risks gives an indication of radiation effects that is generally more meaningful in terms of total social cost than simply cancer deaths alone.

Ascertainment of benign tumors from the tumor registries evidently is somewhat incomplete, as judged by comparison with results obtained from the AHS examinations. Thus it may be that the latter group will yield the most definitive information on benign tumors. It is worth noting that in the AHS, radiation dose-related effects have been observed for nonmalignant thyroid disease, gastric polyps, and uterine fibromas, and in an autopsy study, precancerous breast lesions were also found to be radiation-related.

Confounding Factors

Data concerning host and environmental characteristics such as smoking habits, diet, socioeconomic status, childbearing history, occupation, and many other details have been collected in a series of interview and mail surveys of large subsets of the LSS sample conducted at various times between 1963 and 1981. These data have been useful in efforts to deal with factors other than A-bomb radiation exposure which might affect cancer risks. For example, smoking experience is important to take into account in lung cancer studies, as well as potentially for other smoking-related cancer. Smoking information is available from several of the surveys of the LSS population.

Another important potential confounding factor is exposure of the study population to medical X-rays. Evaluation of this source of additional radiation exposure could be important in future analyses of LSS data, particularly for those subjects given X-ray therapy for benign conditions. A survey of hospitals in the Hiroshima area, as well as among the AHS population, indicates that average cumulative radiation exposure to the bone marrow or gonads since 1945 has been less than 2 rad from diagnostic X-ray, although a few persons in the LSS population have accumulated doses over 20 rad (37). With regard to therapeutic radiation, local doses in excess of 1,000 rad have been received by approximately 2,000 persons in the LSS (33). About 65% of this therapy has been for cancer, therefore among this group the primary interest is in the possibility of second primary malignancies.

Previous Methods of Analysis of LSS Data

Studies of the effects of radiation exposure on mortality and disease incidence in the LSS involve the estimation and comparison of rates, to produce summary measures of risk or to provide detailed descriptions of radiation dose-response. The summary measures reported in most analyses of the LSS data are estimates of absolute excess risk or of relative risk. The absolute risk is the number of excess cases per person year (PY) per rad while the relative risk is the proportional increase in risk per rad. The results in the two cities are age-adjusted to the combined population. Most published analyses of morbidity in the sample have made use of the so-called contingency table method, which was originally developed by Land for a survey of mortality through 1966 (4), and has been used in a slightly modified form in the two recent surveys of mortality in the LSS (5, 23), as well as in special studies of specific diseases, such as Ichimaru et al. (20) and Tokunaga et al. (42). This method has been described in detail by Preston (34). Briefly, statistics for heterogeneity of risk among dose categories are partitioned into sums of squares of asymptotically normal statistics. The latter statistics are simply regression coefficients obtained by the use of orthogonal contrasts designed to test particular alternative hypotheses of interest, an approach derived from Cochran (11). The alternative hypothesis of primary interest has usually been that the radiation-induced absolute excess risk, averaged over some follow-up period of interest, increased as a linear function of radiation exposure dose. The Mantel-Haenszel procedure (28, 29) was employed to calculate expected number of deaths and covariance matrices, adjusting for differences between strata defined by city, sex, and age ATB. The contingency table method, as it has usually been applied in studies at RERF, is based on internal comparisons of mortality rates among exposed survivors. However, some reports (21, 31) have made use of Japanese national death rates for the calculation of expected number of deaths.

The analyses in the various reports cited above were similar in several key respects: 1) In none of the reports were the analyses of trends in dose adjusted for temporal variation of background mortality rates during the period of follow-up. However, recent computations have shown that this adjustment leads to only minor changes in results of analyses of the LSS data. 2) As applied, the contingency table method provided only estimates and test statistics for the radiation dose-response parameter, but did not provide information for formally estimating the magnitude or testing the significance of dose effect modification by other factors. Therefore the comparison of the radiation dose-responses by city, sex, age ATB, or subinterval of follow-up had to be based on informal interpretations of the results of separate analyses for various subsets of the data. An untoward result of this was the necessity for an extremely large number of separate, but frequently correlated significance tests. 3) The observed levels of significance (p values) for the various statistical tests were all based on asymptotic chi-square and normal distributions. For many causes of death, the highly skewed distribution of the LSS sample with respect to radiation dose leads to quite small expected number of deaths in the high dose categories. It has been recognized that in this situation the normal-theory p values underestimate the true significance levels (19). Some reports have attempted to deal with this problem by employing fourth-order Edgeworth approximations of the trend statistic's sampling distributions ($5, 42$).

Historically, retrospective studies have played a less important role than cohort studies for investigations of cancer among A-bomb survivors, although in recent years a number of case-control studies have been undertaken. These have included studies of cancer of the female breast (45), the lung (7), and colon and rectum (1). The procedures and statistical analyses which have been conducted or planned for these case-control studies are based on standard techniques (9) and will not be discussed in this paper.

Hazard Rate Models for the LSS Data

Recent advances in statistical and computational methodology have made it possible to introduce sophisticated and powerful new techniques for the analysis of large sets of survival data. These methods have been described by Cox (13), Kalbfleisch and Prentice (22), Lawless (27), and others. These new techniques, which make use of explicit models for the underlying hazard (instantaneous rate) function make it possible to study the temporal variation in the background and radiogenic components of the observed rates and to formulate and test specific hypotheses about modification of the dose-response by factors such as age ATB and sex. In this section several classes of hazard function models are discussed and some specific models which have proven useful in analyses of the LSS cancer data are described. Computational methods and software for parameter estimation, hypothesis testing, and the assessment of goodness-of-fit based on these models are also discussed briefly. The emphasis here is placed on the case in which there is a single, instantaneous exposure to the factor of primary interest. Thomas (40) and Gilbert (18) consider the use of hazard rate modeling methods in cases of prolonged exposure.

Let $\mu(t; \mathbf{z}, d)$ denote the hazard function at time t for a person who received dose d; the vector $\mathbf{z}$ contains information about covariates other than radiation dose, such as city, sex, age ATB, smoking, etc. The hazard function corresponds to the incidence or mortality rate as a continuous function of time. Two simple models for the hazard function might be considered. In the first, a pure relative risk model, the relative risk is a function of dose only. Such a model can be written as

$$\mu(t; \boldsymbol{z}, d) = \lambda(t; \boldsymbol{z})\rho(d), \tag{1}$$

where $\lambda(t; \boldsymbol{z})$ denotes the natural or background rate of morbidity in the absence of radiation exposure, and $\rho(d)$ is the relative risk function. Similarly, one can define a purely additive excess risk model in which the excess risk for dose d does not depend on time or the other covariates:

$$\mu(t; \boldsymbol{z}, d) = \lambda(t; \boldsymbol{z}) + \varepsilon(d), \tag{2}$$

where $\varepsilon(d)$ is the additive excess risk function. Potentially more realistic models are obtained if we allow for dose-effect modification by the other factors. It is also important to consider more general hazard functions in which the relative and excess risk functions are allowed to vary with time. In their most general form these models can be written as

$$\mu(t; \boldsymbol{z}, d) = \lambda(t; \boldsymbol{z})\rho(d; t, \boldsymbol{z}) \tag{3}$$

and

$$\mu(t; \boldsymbol{z}, d) = \lambda(t; \boldsymbol{z}) + \varepsilon(d; t, \boldsymbol{z}), \tag{4}$$

in which case the distinction between relative and absolute risk models disappears. Useful models for the study of radiation effects lie somewhere between the extremes of the too-simple models (1) and (2) and the too-rich models (3) and (4). In analyses of RERF data based on hazard rate models, excess risks have generally proven to be time dependent. Absolute excess risk models which include such time dependence are generalizations of the standard absolute risk models which are discussed in the literature on radiation effects and which do not allow the excess risk to change in time after an initial latent period; see for example the 1980 BEIR Report (12), 169–172.

In studies at RERF, interest is centered on the dose-related relative or excess risk functions. Partial likelihood methods for relative risk models, as originally proposed by Cox (13) and discussed at length by Kalbfleisch and Prentice (22), allow one to focus on the estimation of the relative risk without the explicit estimation of the background hazard function $\lambda(t; \boldsymbol{z})$. It is sometimes of interest in relative risk models, and it is necessary for estimation in absolute excess risk models, to consider fully specified parametric models for the background rates (*i.e.*, the natural rates of mortality or disease incidence in the absence of exposure to radiation). The models used for background rates in current studies at RERF are generally log-linear models of the form $\exp(\beta^{*}\boldsymbol{z}^{*})$ where $\boldsymbol{z}^{*}$ includes not only variables related to city, sex, smoking, *etc.*, but also functions of attained age which replace the time-since-exposure variable t. Continuous or indicator functions of age ATB can be included to allow for secular trends in the rates.

Discussions of relative risk functions are often based on log-linear ($e\beta\boldsymbol{x}$) or additive $(1+\beta\boldsymbol{x})$ forms for the relative risk, where the vector $\boldsymbol{x}=x(d, \boldsymbol{z})$ can include both dose- and covariate-related components. A simple example of the former is β, while an example of the latter is given by $(1+\beta, \beta+\boldsymbol{z})$ where $\boldsymbol{z}$ is a potential dose effect modifier such as a function of age ATB.

Recently there has been interest in general relative risk models which can be used to discriminate between multiplicative and additive relative risks. Aranda-Ordaz (2) and Breslow (8) have suggested the use of relative risk functions of the form

$$l(\rho(\boldsymbol{x})) = [(1+\beta\boldsymbol{x})^{\delta}-1]/\delta \tag{5}$$

This class of relative risk models includes both the multiplicative and additive models as special cases; $\delta=1$ for the multiplicative and the limit as δ goes to 0 for the additive model. Thomas (41) has suggested an alternative approach to this problem.

The excess risk models used thus far in analyses of the A-bomb survivor data have the form

$$\varepsilon(d, \mathbf{z}) = \phi(d)\omega(\mathbf{z}, t)$$

where the $\phi(d)$ is typically linear in dose and $\omega(t, \mathbf{z})$ is log-linear in various functions of the covariates and time. The function $\phi(d)$ can be thought of as a baseline dose-response while the function $\omega(t, \mathbf{z})$ allows for deviations from this baseline dose-response due to characteristics of the individuals or the passage of time. While the baseline dose-response can be linear, one could easily consider nonlinear functions of total dose.

Methods of Estimation for Hazard Rate Models

Likelihood methods are used for parameter estimation and hypothesis testing with hazard rate models. A few analyses have been carried out using the full likelihood for the ungrouped data. Such analyses have been done primarily to compare the resulting parameter estimates and their standard errors with those obtained when functionally identical models were fit to grouped data using the methods outlined below. Full likelihood methods are not practical for use with general, time-dependent hazard rate models such as those described above.

Partial likelihood methods for relative risk models have proven useful in the analysis of the RERF data. As noted above, this approach is appealing because it eliminates the need to model the background rates explicitly. Although partial likelihood methods cannot be used for absolute risk models, the inclusion of time-dependent covariates makes it possible to consider relative risks which are not constant in time. The major limitation of this approach is that it is computationally intensive. On a medium-sized mainframe computer (*e.g.*, NEC ACOS-450) over one hour of computer time is required to fit a relative risk model with time-dependent covariates to the LSS data.

Another approach to the analysis of large sets of survival data which overcomes the limitations of the methods discussed above makes use of grouped data. The ideas underlying the use of grouped data in the analysis of cohort studies have been described in several recent papers (8, 10, 17, 32). As in the contingency table analysis described above, the basic data are the number of cases or deaths, Y_{ijk}, and PY or number of persons at risk, P_{ijk}, together with a dose, d_{ij}, and vector of covariates, $\mathbf{z}_{ijk}$, associated with each cell in a cross-classification over city, sex, age ATB, and, perhaps, other factors (i), dose groups (j), and subintervals of follow-up (k). The components of $\mathbf{z}_{ijk}$ may be indicator variables or, for quantitative factors such as age, time, cigarette consumption, *etc.*, classmark values such as category-specific means or midpoints; the components of $\mathbf{z}_{ijk}$ may also include cross-products involving dose. If the P_{ijk} are regarded as fixed and the risk per unit time is considered to be a constant, μ_{ijk}, within each cell of the cross-classification, then the kernel of the likelihood function is identical to that which would arise if the Y_{ijk} are treated as independent Poisson random variables with mean $P_{ijk}\mu_{ijk}$. The parameters μ_{ijk} correspond to specific rates of incidence or mortality. For the purpose of modelling these rates, parametric or semiparametric models for the underlying hazard function can be considered. Maximum likelihood estimation and likelihood-based hypothesis tests are derived from the Poisson likelihood.

This approach has many advantages. First, it can be used to fit either relative risk or absolute excess risk models. The theory of likelihood-based inference provides a variety of standard techniques for hypothesis testing and estimation (*14*). For example, it is possible to compute confidence intervals for complex functions of hazard rate such as absolute excess risk, relative risk, or attributable risk at a given time or averaged over a specific period of follow-up. Also, since the likelihood is identical to a Poisson likelihood, the computations for many hazard rate models can be performed using standard programs for Poisson regression. As noted by Frome (*17*) and others, regression diagnostics can be used to assess the influence of individual points or groups of points on the fitted models. Alternatively, one can examine the patterns of standardized residuals in marginal subtables formed by full or partial collapsing of the cross-classification over one or more dimensions.

It is practical to use interactive programs for parameter estimation and model comparison since the reduction of the data by grouping greatly reduces the computational burdens, especially for models with time dependent covariates. Parameter estimation for many hazard function models can easily be carried out with the generalized linear interactive modelling program GLIM (*3*), which is widely available. The use of GLIM for hazard function modelling is particularly simple if the hazard function is assumed to be a log-linear function of time, dose, and the other covariates. GLIM can also be used for parameter estimation in more general models with user-defined macros. Virtually all of the work on the absolute excess risk models for leukemia incidence described by Pierce *et al.* (*32*) was carried out by means of GLIM macros.

For general use in analyses at RERF, an interactive computer program, AMFIT, has been developed. This program can be used for unconditional maximum likelihood estimation in a wide variety of relative and excess risk models. One feature of AMFIT is the use of an algorithm (*16*) for the estimation of multiplicative strata parameters. This algorithm makes it possible to fit hazard rate models of the form

$$\mu_{ijk} = \lambda_{ij}\rho(d_{ij}, \mathbf{z}_{ijk}) \tag{6}$$

in which a separate multiplicative parameter, λ_{ik}, is estimated for each of a large number of strata without the need to invert large matrices: the size of the matrix to be inverted at each iteration depends only upon the number of parameters in the relative risk function and not on the number of strata parameters. AMFIT can also be used for parameter estimation with the general relative risk function given in model (6). Details regarding the design and usage of AMFIT are available from RERF and will be published elsewhere. Examples of analyses of RERF data which make use of the general hazard rate models available in AMFIT include studies of the incidence of leukemia (*32*) and lung cancer (*26*), as well as studies, currently in progress, of the incidence of thyroid cancer and of general mortality in the LSS sample.

Conditional maximum likelihood methods can also be used to estimate parameters associated with the relative risk function in model (5). The PECAN program (*39*) can be used for this purpose. Unconditional maximum likelihood methods such as those available in PECAN are particularly useful in the analysis of case-control studies.

CONCLUSION

During the past few decades at Atomic Bomb Casualty Commission (ABCC)-RERF, much has been learned about radiation carcinogenesis from studies of the LSS sample, various subsamples such as the AHS, and additional study samples such as the in utero exposed group. The major study samples and data collection systems were established in the 1950s and were designed to make the best possible use of the human and technological resources available at that time. Once established, these samples and systems have remained basically unchanged to the present time and have, in general, functioned well.

Recent years have seen profound improvements in statistical methods for the analysis of epidemiologic data. The introduction of such methods has provided powerful techniques for detailed investigations of the excess risks associated with exposure to ionizing radiation. In particular the potential exists for more thorough study of important questions about interactions between the effects of radiation and other factors such as age at exposure or sex. The time course of radiation effects can also be studied in more detail than was previously possible.

The power of these recently developed statistical methods notwithstanding, it is important to realize that the extent to which the long-term effects of exposure to A-bomb radiation will be understood adequately is determined to a large extent by the quantity and quality of the available data. Although the LSS sample is large and has experienced a large number of cancer incident cases and deaths, the number of excess cancer cases attributable to A-bomb radiation exposure will remain rather small. For leukemia, with about 90 out of 220 deaths attributable to radiation exposure, adequate statistical power is available for detailed inferences concerning the radiation dose-response, its time course, and modification of the dose-response by other factors such as age ATB. Similar considerations apply to other cancer types of comparable radiosensitivity. For some cancer, however, the excess attributable to radiation will be much smaller, which makes it difficult in these instances to reach precise inferences about second-order effects such as interactions between radiation and age ATB or the time course of the radiation dose-response.

Much remains to be learned about the effects of exposure to A-bomb radiation. The adoption of a dosimetry system to replace the T65 dose estimates will necessitate careful reevaluation of all aspects of the radiation dose-response. The potential exists for profound changes in currently held notions of human radiation carcinogenesis as the youngest members of the LSS sample reach the ages of greatest cancer risk. It is essential that RERF, with an awareness of both the strengths and weaknesses of its data resources, continually seek the highest possible quality of epidemiologic and statistical methodology.

REFERENCES

1. Akiba, S., Land, C. E., Kinlen, L. J., Ershow, S., Nakatsuka, H., and Sekine, I. A case-control study on colorectal cancer. RERF Res. Protoc. 6-83 (1983).
2. Aranda-Ordaz, F. J. An extension of the proportional hazards model for grouped data. *Biometrics*, **39**, 109–117 (1983).
3. Baker, R. J. and Nelder, J. A. The GLIM System: Release 3. Numerical Algorithms Group, Oxford (1978).
4. Beebe, G. W., Kato, H., and Land, C. E. Studies of the mortality of A-bomb survivors. 4. Mortality and radiation dose, 1950–1966. *Radiat. Res.*, **48**, 613–649 (1971).
5. Beebe, G. W., Kato, H., and Land, C. E. Studies of the mortality of a A-bomb survivors. 6. Mortality and radiation dose, 1950–1974. *Radiat. Res.*, **75**, 138–201 (1978).
6. Beebe, G. W. and Usagawa, M. The major RERF samples. ABCC Tech. Rep. 12-68 (1968).
7. Blot, W. J., Akiba, S., and Kato H. Ionizing radiation and lung cancer: a review including

preliminary results from a case-control study among A-bomb survivors. *In* "Atomic Bomb Survivor Data: Utilization and Analysis," ed. R. L. Prentice and D. J. Thompson, pp. 235–248 (1984). SIAM, Philadelphia.

8. Breslow, N. E. Cohort analysis in epidemiology. University of Washington, Dept. of Biostatistics. Technical Report No. 65 (1984).

9. Breslow, N. E. and Day, N. E. "Statistical Methods in Cancer Research Volume 1—The Analysis of Case-control Studies (1980). IARC, Lyon.

10. Breslow, N. E., Lubin, J. H., Marek, P., and Langholz, B. Multiplicative models and cohort analysis. *J. Am. Stat. Assoc.*, **78**, 1–12 (1983).

11. Cochran, W. G. Some methods for strengthening the common x2 tests. *Biometrics*, **10**, 417–451 (1954).

12. Committee on the Biological Effects of Ionizing Radiation. The Effects on Populations of Exposure to Low Levels of Ionizing Radiation: 1980 (1980) National Academy Press, Washington, D.C.

13. Cox, D. R. Regression models and life tables (with discussion). *J. R. Stat. Soc. Ser. B*, **34**, 187–220 (1972).

14. Cox, D. R. and Hinkley, D. V. "Theoretical Statistics" (1974). Methuen, New York.

15. Daiwa Health Foundation. Atlas of cancer mortality for Japan by cities and counties, 1969–71, Tokyo, 1977.

16. Dempster, A. P., Laird, N. M., and Rubin, D. B. Maximum likelihood from incomplete data *via* the Em algorithm. *J. R. Stat. Soc. Ser. B.*, **39**, 1–38 (1977).

17. Frome, E. L. The analysis of rates using Poisson regression models. *Biometrics*, **39**, 665–674 (1983).

18. Gilbert, E. S. An evaluation of several methods for assessing the effects of occupational exposure to radiation. *Biometrics*, **39**, 161–171 (1983).

19. Hoel, D. G. and Jennrich, R. I. Life table analysis with small numbers of cases, an example multiple myeloma in Hiroshima and Nagasaki. RERF Tech. Rep. 9–84 (1984).

20. Ichimaru, M., Ishimaru, T., Mikami, M., Yamada, Y., and Ohkita, T. Incidence of leukemia in a fixed cohort of atomic bomb survivors and controls, Hiroshima and Nagasaki: October 1950—December 1978. RERF Tech. Rep. 13-81 (1981).

21. Jablon, S. and Kato, H. Studies of the mortality of A-bomb survivors. 5. Radiation dose and mortality, 1950–1970. *Radiat. Res.* **50**, 649–698 (1972).

22. Kalbfleisch, J. D. and Prentice, R. L. "The Statistical Analysis of Failure Time Data" (1980). Wiley, New York.

23. Kato, H. and Schull, W. J. Studies of the mortality of the A-bomb survivors. 7. Mortality 1950–1978, Part I. Cancer Mortality. *Radiat. Res.*, **90**, 395–432 (1982).

24. Kerr, G. D., Pace, J. V., III, and Scott, W. H., Jr. Tissue kerma *vs.* distance relationships for initial nuclear radiation from the atomic bombs, Hiroshima and Nagasaki (1983). *In* "Reassessment of Atomic Bomb Dosimetry," pp. 57–103. (1983) RERF, Hiroshima.

25. Kodama, K., Shimizu, Y., Sawada, H., and Kato, H. Incidence of stroke and coronary heart disease in the Adult Health Study sample, 1958–78. RERF Tech. Rep. 22-84 (1984).

26. Kopecky, K. J., Yamamoto, T., Fujikura, T., Tokuoka, S., Monzen, T., Nishimori, I., Nakashima, E., and Kato, H. Lung cancer, radiation exposure and smoking among atomic bomb survivors, Hiroshima and Nagasaki, 1950–1980. RERF Tech. Rep. in preparation.

27. Lawless, J. F. "Statistical Models and Methods for Lifetime Data" (1982). Wiley, New York.

28. Mantel, N. and Haenszel, W. Statistical aspects of the analysis of data from retrospective studies of disease. *J. Natl. Cancer Inst.*, **22**, 719–748 (1959).

29. Mantel, N. Chi-square tests with one degree of freedom: extensions of the Mantel-Haenszel procedure. *J. Am. Stat. Assoc.*, **58**, 690–700 (1963).

30. Milton, R. C. and Shohoji, T. Tentative 1965 radiation dose estimation for A-bomb survivors, Hiroshima and Nagasaki, ABCC Tech. Rep. 1-68 (1968).

31. Moriyama, I. M. and Kato, H. JNIH-ABCC Life Span Study, Report 7. Mortality experience of A-bomb survivors, 1950–72. ABCC Tech. Rep. 15-73 (1973).

32. Pierce, D. A., Preston, D. L., and Ishimaru, T. A method of analysis of cancer incidence in Japanese atomic bomb survivors with application to acute leukemia, RERF Tech. Rep. 15-83 (1983).

33. Pinkston, J. A., Antoku, S., and Russell, W. J. Malignant neoplasms among atomic bomb survivors following radiation therapy. *Acta Radiol. Oncol.*, **20**, 267–271 (1981). (Also personal communication, W. J. Russell, 1984).

34. Preston, D. L. Cancer mortality and incidence in the Life Span Study: statistical methods used in Reports Five through Ten. *In* "Atomic Bomb Survivor Data: Utilization and Analysis," ed. R. L. Prentice and D. J. Thompson, pp. 35–50 (1984). SIAM, Philadelphia.

35. Radford, E. P. A comparison of incidence and mortality as a basis for determining risks from environmental agents. *In* "Proc. of the 20th Annual Meeting of the National Council on Radiation Protection and Measurements," pp. 75–88 (1985). NCRP, Bethesda, Md.

36. Sawada, H., Kodama, K., Shimizu, Y., and Kato, H. RERF Adult Health Study Report 6: Results of six examination cycles, 1968–1980. Hiroshima and Nagasaki. RERF Tech. Rep., in preparation.

37. Sawada, W., Land, C. E., Otake, M., Russell, W. J., Takeshita, K., Yoshinaga, H., and Hombo, Z. Hospital and clinic survey estimates of medical x-ray exposures in Hiroshima and Nagasaki. Part I, RERF population and the general population. RERF Tech. Rep. 16-79 (1979).

38. Steer, A., Moriyama, I. M., and Shimizu, K. The autopsy program and the life span study, January 1951–December, 1970. ABCC Tech. Rep. 16-73 (1973).

39. Storer, B. E., Wacholder, S., and Breslow, N. E. Maximum likelihood fitting of general risk models to stratified data. *Appl. Stat.*, **32**, 177–181 (1983).

40. Thomas, D. C. General relative risk models for survival time and matched case-control analysis. *Biometrics*, **37**, 673–686 (1981).

41. Thomas, D. C. Temporal effects and interactions in cancer: Implications of carcinogenic models. *In* "Environmental Health: Risk Assessment," ed. R. L. Prentice and A. S. Whittemore, pp. 107–121 (1982). SIAM, Philadelphia.

42. Tokunaga, M., Land, C. E., Yamamoto, T., Asano, M., Tokuoka, S., Ezaki, H., and Nishimori, I. Incidence of female breast cancer among atomic bomb survivors, Hiroshima and Nagasaki, 1950–80. RERF Tech. Rep. 15-84 (1984).

43. Wakabayashi, T., Kato, H., Ideda, T., and Schull, W. J. Studies of the mortality of A-bomb survivors, Report 7. Part III. Incidence of cancer in 1959–78, based on the Tumor Registry data, Nagasaki. *Radiat. Res.*, **93**, 112–146 (1983).

44. Woolson, W. A., Gritzner, M. L., and Egbert, S. D. Atomic bomb survivor dosimetry. Report to RERF, Dec. 1984.

45. Yamada, Y., Land, C. E., and Hayakawa, N. Interaction between radiation dose and host factors. An epidemiological case-control study of female breast cancer in atomic bomb survivors. RERF Res. Protoc. 14-79 (1979).

46. Yamamoto, T., Moriyama, I. M., Asano, M., and Guralnick, L. The Autopsy Program and the Life Span Study, January 1961–December 1975. RERF Tech. Rep. 18-78 (1978).

GANN Monograph on Cancer Research 32, 1986

EXPERIMENTAL RADIATION CARCINOGENESIS IN RODENTS

Kenjiro YOKORO, Toshio SEYAMA, and Kazuyoshi YANAGIHARA

*Department of Pathology, Research Institute for Nuclear Medicine and Biology, Hiroshima University**

Leukemia, lymphoma, and mammary tumors induced in rodents by ionizing radiation appear, in many aspects, to be the counterparts to those in man as have been observed among the atomic-bomb (A-bomb) survivors.

The emphasis of radiation-induced leukemogenesis was placed on the induction of lymphoid leukemia originating in the thymus (thymic lymphoma), which is most frequently encountered in irradiated mice. In addition to the well-defined factors governing the development and progression of the disease, recent developing interest on the etiological implication of retroviruses and cellular oncogenes is also discussed.

Radiation-induced mammary carcinogenesis in rats is a suitable model for study of human breast cancer with regard to their hormone responsiveness. Our experimental observations using various radiations with different energies in combination with prolactin are described, emphasizing the key role of the promotion phase in carcinogenesis. The experimental system enabled us to demonstrate a high relative biological effectiveness (RBE) of fission spectrum neutrons, which may indicate strong contribution of fission neutrons in induction of malignant tumors among survivors.

The principal late effect of ionizing radiation is the development of cancer in various tissues of man and animals. Among these, leukemia-lymphoma and mammary tumors are most frequently encountered in certain species including man as evidenced by observations in atomic bomb (A-bomb) survivors. In this report, therefore, the description will be limited to these two neoplasms induced in experimental animals by exposure to ionizing radiation; leukemia-lymphoma in mice is reviewed at some length, giving emphasis to the induction mechanism, and mammary tumors in rats in a brief manner calling attention to the high relative biological effectiveness of fission spectrum neutrons.

I. RADIATION-INDUCED LEUKEMOGENESIS IN MICE

Introduction and Historical Background

Leukemia is one of the best known neoplasms causally related to radiation exposure both in man and animals. The first report by Van Jagic *et al.* (*128*) on the leukemogenic effect of radiation in man has been amply confirmed by many investigators (*24, 97, 123*). These early findings in man and data accumulated for experimental animals enabled

---

* Kasumi 1-2-3, Minami-ku, Hiroshima 734, Japan (横路謙次郎, 瀬山敏雄, 柳原五吉).

experts to predict that an excess incidence of leukemia and other neoplasms would occur among survivors exposed to atomic radiation in Hiroshima and Nagasaki (*1*).

Although experimental studies on radiation-induced leukemogenesis have been pursued in several animal species, studies in mice have been most fruitful in producing many valuable insights into leukemogenesis. This review will deal, then, with radiogenic leukemia in mice. The leukemogenic effect of ionizing radiation in mice was first demonstrated in the early 1930s independently by Krebs *et al.* (*80*), Hueper (*49*), and Furth and Furth (*22*). These investigators observed the development of various types of leukemia in X-irradiated mice with a several-fold increased incidence compared to that in non-irradiated controls. Among these pioneers, Furth and Furth (*22*) described not only the induction of leukemia, but also that of other solid neoplastic lesions in three different irradiated mouse strains, thus demonstrating the powerful tumorigenic potency of ionizing radiation.

In the meantime, Furth (*19*) and Furth *et al.* (25) succeeded in establishing a mouse strain, Ak (presently known as AKR) in which lymphoma or lymphoid leukemia, originating mainly in the thymus, occurs spontaneously at a high rate before reaching one year of age. The viral nature of Ak leukemia was later shown by Gross (*27, 28*) who isolated a leukemogenic type-C RNA virus from leukemic tissue (passage A virus of Gross).

The leukemogenic potency of certain chemicals (*8, 23*) and of estrogenic hormones (*82*) in mice was also demonstrated in the 1930s. Thus, such agents as radiation, chemicals, hormones, and virus, presently recognized as leukemogens had already been discovered more than four decades ago.

The epoch-making discoveries in leukemia research are as follows:

1.   Recognition of leukemogenic potency of radiation, chemicals, and hormones. Furth and Furth (1936), Krebs *et al.* (1930), Hueper (1934), Burrows and Cook (1936), Furth and Furth (1938), Lacassagne (1937).

2.   Creation of a high leukemic mouse strain, Ak (AKR), and isolation of a leukemogenic virus from Ak lymphoma. Furth *et al.* (1933), Gross (1951).

3.   Demonstration of "indirect induction mechanism" in radiation leukemogenesis, and isolation of a leukemogenic virus (Radiation Leukemia Virus, Rad LV) from radiation-induced lymphoma of C57BL/Ka mice. Kaplan *et al.* (1956), Lieberman and Kaplan (1959).

4.   Isolation of leukemogenic viruses from transplantable, solid mouse tumors, such as Friend, Graffi, Moloney, and Rauscher viruses.

5.   Proposal of "oncogene hypothesis"; concept of endogenous RNA viruses, and their role in leukemogenesis. Huebner and Todaro (1969).

6.   Role of recombinant virus (mink cell focus-inducing, MCF virus) in leukemogenesis; mode of its involvement Hartley *et al.* (1977), Lee and Ihle (1979), Hayward *et al.* (1981), Fischinger *et al.* (1982), Tress *et al.* (1982), Rassart *et al.* (1983).

Type of Leukemia

1.   Thymic lymphoma (localized and generalized)

This type of lymphoma (leukemia), originating in the thymus, is far more frequently encountered than the other types of leukemia in many common mouse strains following exposure to ionizing radiation. A high incidence of thymic lymphoma with a short latent period can be obtained by appropriately fractionated whole-body irradiation rather than with a single dose (*69*). A detailed histological study (*115*) revealed that the disease may be initiated unilaterally in an atrophic lobe, followed by invasion into the other lobe, and later forming a huge tumor mass occupying the thoracic cavity. The localized lymphoma eventually disseminates into the visceral organs and the peripheral blood becomes leukemic, the form of which may be the counterpart of acute lymphoid leukemia in children. The tumor cells are morphologically lymphoblastic and carry a cell surface antigen (Thy. 1) which is specific for the T lymphocyte.

2. *Granulocytic (myeloid) leukemia*

Myeloid leukemia in mice, developing either spontaneously or induced by leukemogenic agents, is much less commonly encountered and has been less extensively studied than lymphoid leukemia. The RF (RFM, RF/Jax) strain of mice, originally developed by Furth (*19*) as a low leukemic strain, is a remarkable exception. Upton *et al.* (*124–126*) and Hiraki *et al.* (*44*) reported that myeloid leukemia developed in as high as 40%–50% of young adult male RF mice following a single exposure to 150–450 rad of X-rays. However, in a later study, a much lower incidence of myeloid leukemia was reported in irradiated RF mice maintained under a special pathogen-free condition (*122*). The latent period was slightly longer than that of thymic lymphoma; a majority of cases appeared between 5 to 18 months after irradiation. Myeloid leukemia is characterized by the development of prominent splenomegaly and the appearance of immature granulocytic cells in the peripheral blood. The thymus is usually atrophic. In some cases, leukemic tissue exhibits a yellowish-green color, which is considered to be the counterpart of chloroma or chloroleukemia in man. The disease should be distinguished from leukemoid reaction which is accompanied by infections or amyloidosis.

3. *Nonthymic lymphoma and reticulum cell sarcoma*

These tumors occur much later in life than other types of leukemias. The influence of radiation in induction of nonthymic lymphoma has not been clearly demonstrated, although an increased incidence has been observed in thymectomized mice following exposure to single whole-body irradiation (*124*). RF mice exposed to a single dose of irradiation, either gamma rays or neutrons, show a decrease in the incidence of reticulum cell sarcoma (*122*).

Stemming from the mouse system, modern lymphocytology now contributes much to the progress of fundamental and clinical medicine. The present classification of mouse leukemia is based mainly on the morphology of leukemic cells. A new classification based not only the morphological but also immunological characteristics should be introduced as has been attempted in the human system.

Factors Influencing Radiation-induced Leukemogenesis

It has been well documented that the induction pattern of radiogenic leukemia is modified to a large extent by radiological, physiological, and environmental factors. Kaplan and his associates at Stanford University, who used C57BL/Ka mice as the model system, have made many contributions to the fundamental knowledge of radiogenic thymic lymphoma (*63, 65*). Studies conducted on RF mice by Upton (*124*) and currently by Ullrich *et al.* (*121*) have furnished a great deal of information on myeloid leukemia.

1.   Radiological factors

A)   Dose and dose rate

Exposure of 4 to 5 week old C57BL mice to fractionated whole-body X-irradiation (four exposures of 150–170 rad each at 5–8 day intervals is most efficient for inducing thymic lymphoma, resulting in the development of lymphomas in about 70%–90% of mice with a mean latent period of about 180 days. This procedure may also be applicable to most other strains.

In male RF mice, a single whole-body X-irradiation of 150, 300 and 450 rad resulted in the development of myeloid leukemia in 34%, 38%, and 23%, respectively, while those of thymic lymphoma were 5%, 16%, and 21%, respectively, indicating the absence of dose-dependency for myeloid leukemia and its presence for thymic lymphoma (*124*). In similarly irradiated specific-pathogen-free RF mice, however, a lower incidence of myeloid leukemia and an increased incidence of thymic lymphoma was observed as compared with previously reported data in the conventional counterparts (*122*).

With respect to the effect of dose rate, leukemia inductivity by low linear energy transfer (LET) radiation (X-ray or gamma ray) appears to be much dependent on the dose rate (*e.g.*, a lower dose rate results in a lower incidence) whereas that by high LET radiation (neutrons) is rather independent of it (*93, 121, 126*).

B)   Single vs. fractionated exposure

Fractionated whole-body irradiation with appropriate dose and interval has been proven to be most efficient in induction of thymic lymphoma, whereas dose fractionation seems to have little influence in the case of myeloid leukemia (*68, 127*). Generally speaking, however, the induction rate of myeloid leukemia has never exceeded that of thymic lymphoma using presently available procedures. There appear to be some barriers to overcome that limit the prevalence of radiogenic myeloid leukemia. Since the latent period of myeloid leukemia is longer than that of thymic lymphoma, some of the irradiated mice which might have developed myeloid leukemia will succumb to thymic lymphoma or to other intercurrent diseases before myeloid leukemia develops. The introduction of both a new means and a more susceptible mouse strain is desired for better understanding of the pathogenesis of myeloid leukemia.

C)   Whole-body vs. partial-body irradiation

Whole-body irradiation is essential for efficient induction of thymic lymphoma; irradiation of either the upper or lower half of the body drastically reduces the induction rate. Inhibition of lymphoma development is also achieved by such procedures as lead shielding of the exteriorized spleen, the thigh, and the thymus during irradiation (*60, 66, 95*). These observations suggest a complex mechanism for lymphomagenesis. The incidence of myeloid leukemia in RF mice was also decreased by partial-body shielding (*124*).

D)   Induction of leukemia by radioactive nuclides

Experimental induction of leukemia in mice by radioactive nuclides (internal emitters) has been studied much less extensively than external irradiation.

Brues *et al.* (*7*) might be the first who showed the leukemogenic effect of radiophosphorus (^{32}P) in mice. Hormberg *et al.* (*46, 47*) reported that in BALB mice, the incidence of leukemia is increased following administration of ^{32}P and that leukemias so induced are transmissible by leukemic-cell-free extracts. They also demonstrated the presence of A- and C-type viral particles in leukemic tissue. These observations led them to speculate about the implication of a viral agent in the induction mechanism. A fractionated intraperitoneal injection of ^{32}P (0.5 μCi/mouse, twice a week for 5 weeks, totalling about 100 to 150 μCi/mouse) resulted in the development of thymic lymphomas in 80% of RF/Jax mice. The incidence was substantially reduced by the removal of both the thymus and spleen prior to ^{32}P treatment. Ito *et al.* (*55*) and Takizawa *et al.* (*117*) observed a prevalence of nonthymic stem cell leukemia and reticulum cell leukemia as well as osteogenic sarcomas following a single i.p. injection of radiostrontium (^{90}Sr, 10 μCi/g body weight), the incidence of which was almost comparable with that of thymic lymphomas in mice exposed to fractionated X-irradiation. At the present time, not much information is available as to the most efficient means of leukemia induction by internal emitters.

2. Genetic and physiological factors

A) Strain and age

It has been well established that the frequency of lymphoma development among low-leukemic strains of mice is readily increased to varying degrees of susceptibility of 25%–90% by whole-body exposure to ionizing radiation (*31, 55, 69*). The susceptibility of RF mice to the development of radiogenic myeloid leukemia has been well documented, but relatively less is known for other strains. Fractionated irradiation started at 3–5 weeks of age is most effective for thymic lymphoma induction, and the induction rate decreases rapidly as starting age advances (*58, 59*). It has been shown that, in certain mouse strains, the susceptibility for thymic lymphoma development is maximal when irradiated at birth (*114, 124*). In contrast, the induction rate of myeloid leukemia in RF mice is not much influenced by advancing the age up to at least 6 months.

B) Sex

Development of radiogenic thymic lymphoma predominates in female and myeloid leukemia is more common in males of both C57BL and RF strains. Ovariectomy or orchidectomy has little effect on the induction rate of either type of leukemia (*61, 124*). However, administration of estrogen together with irradiation promoted the development of thymic lymphoma while administration of androgen inhibited it (*67, 78, 118, 132*). Ullrich and Storer (*122*) stated that in RF mice exposed to various single doses of gamma rays, there were no significant differences between female and male dose-response relationships when the incidence of all types of leukemia was examined.

C) Effect of thymectomy and splenectomy

Thymectomy prior to or shortly after irradiation practically eliminates the development of lymphoma, while it has no effect on myeloid leukemia (*61*). On the other hand, splenectomy is highly effective in reducing myeloid leukemia, but has little or no effect on thymic lymphoma (*124*).

3. Immunological capability

It is logical to anticipate that exposure to radiation, in addition to its leukemogenic property, may create favorable conditions for the development and progression of leukemia through its immunosuppressive effect (*38*). However, the role of immunological capability of the irradiated host in facilitating the leukemogenic process has not yet been elucidated. Ito *et al.* (*54*) observed a long standing suppression of both humoral and cellular immune responses in ICR/JCL mice following leukemogenic fractionated X-irradiation, whereas i.p. injection of a leukemogenic dose of ^{90}Sr rather heightened the humoral immune response. Haran-Ghera (*35*) stated that the transient immune impairment following fractionated irradiation does not seem to contribute to the proliferation of preleukemic cells, and Sado (*112*) also showed that the function of T-cell subsets of B10BR mice has been little affected by leukemogenic fractionated X-irradiation.

Recently, it was reported that leukemogenic irradiation resulted in severe depression of spontaneous natural killer (NK) cell activity, that the activity could be restored by bone marrow transplantation from nonirradiated mice (*108*). Moreover, the development of radiogenic lymphomas is significantly inhibited by the injection of a "cloned cell line with NK activity" shortly after irradiation (*131*). The role of NK activity in T-cell leukemogenesis deserves further exploration.

4.   *Influence of microbial environment*

The induction rate of radiogenic myeloid leukemia has been generally higher (*124*) in RF mice kept in conventional laboratory conditions than in mice maintained in a specific-pathogen-free state (*122*). The reason for the difference is not clear, but it is conceived that either the number of myeloid stem cells at risk or their proliferative rate might be dependent on the microbial environment (*18*). The reverse is true for the induction of thymic lymphoma; viral or bacterial infections may cause thymic involution that may lead the thymus to be less responsive to lymphoma development.

5.   *Hematolymphopoietic factors*

The fact that partial-body shielding is effective in reducing the rate of thymic lymphoma (*66*) and that local irradiation to the thymus is likewise ineffective, raise the question as to whether or not there is a direct lymphomagenic effect of radiation on the target tissue, the thymus. It was soon shown that intravenous injection of normal, but not of preirradiated bone marrow cells or spleen homogenates shortly after leukemogenic doses of irradiation substantially reduced the incidence of thymic lymphoma (*72*). These procedures, by which lymphoma incidence is reduced, are also shown to accelerate the regenerative process of the radiation-injured thymus.

It was concluded (*96*), though there was some admittedly conflicting evidence, that the effect of bone marrow transplantation in reducing lymphoma incidence, as well as saving lethally-irradiated mice (*12, 94*), was attributable to the repopulation of hematolymphopoietic tissues by the injected cellular component, but not to a humoral factor. These findings emphasize that the inseparable relation of the bone marrow and thymus under both physiologically normal and pathological conditions is now indisputably established.

Role of the Thymus and Bone Marrow

1.   *Induction of thymic lymphoma*

The role of the thymus and bone marrow, and their interaction in T-cell lymphomagenesis has been discussed at length by several investigators (*35, 63, 102*). The majority of T-cell lymphomas developing either spontaneously or following leukemogenic treatment is initiated in the thymus, and thymectomy practically eliminates the occurrence of the disease (*61, 85, 86, 89, 99*). Observations of Law and Miller (*85*) that thymectomy was effective in lowering spontaneous lymphoma in C58 mice, of which about 50% are of nonthymic origin, led them to point out that an explanation for effects other than removal of potentially malignant cells by thymectomy is needed. Law and Miller (*86*) also found that autoplastic grafting of the thymus restored the susceptibility of thymectomized mice to carcinogen-induced lymphomagenesis, indicating that the presence of the thymus is a prerequisite to the development of lymphoma.

A series of experiments by Kaplan and his associates (9, 70, 71, 73, 74) demonstrated that the susceptibility of thymectomized mice to radiation-induced lymphomagenesis is restored by subcutaneous implantation of the thymus derived from newborn syngeneic mice. Furthermore, it was shown by Kaplan et al. and by Law and Potter (87) that a certain proportion of lymphomas, which developed at the site of the neonatal thymus graft in thymectomized-irradiated mice were, indeed, nonirradiated donor cell in origin. The finding was recently reconfirmed (103).

This indirect induction mechanism together with findings described in the preceding section motivated investigators to speculate that whole-body irradiation inactivates an anti-leukemic factor in the body or activates a latent leukemogenic virus. Similar experiments in rats conducted in this laboratory appeared to support the idea (137).

From the preceding findings, it is clear that concurrent injury to both bone marrow and thymus by whole-body irradiation is essential for the efficient induction of radiogenic thymic lymphoma. Other leukemogens such as urethane and 7, 12-dimethylbenz (a) anthracene (DMBA) also produce a similar effect in susceptible mice (37, 110). It has been shown that the regenerative process of the thymus in whole-body irradiated mice is retarded (maturation arrest), as indicated by the persistence of large immature cells in the depleted cortex. These immature cells have been considered to be the target of leukemogenesis (63). Some investigators stress the importance of population changes of blastic cells in both bone marrow and thymus during radiation-induced lymphomagenesis (6).

Where, then, are these cells derived from and when does malignant transformation take place? Haran-Ghera (35, 36) at Weizmann Institute, demonstrated in C57BL/6 mice with an ingenious transplantation assay method (21) the existence of potentially malignant cells, not of the T-cell phenotype (36), in the bone marrow but not in the thymus or in the spleen, within 30 days after termination of leukemogenic fractionated irradiation, that is to say, long before the occurrence of frank lymphoma when Thy. 1 antigen is expressed on the cell surface. It is of interest that procedures known to lower the lymphoma incidence, such as partial shielding, bone marrow transplantation, or thymectomy did not reduce the occurrence of preleukemic cells in the marrow. These results strongly suggest that radiation-induced cell transformation takes place in the bone marrow, rather than in the thymus. On the other hand, a recent report of the Stanford group (5) suggested that the primary site of neoplastic transformation in irradiated C57BL/Ka mice is the thymus rather than the bone marrow, which is at variance with the findings of Haran-Ghera (37). It appears that opinions among investigators do not coincide with each other and are rather confusing as to the interaction of the bone marrow and the thymus. At any rate, radiation-transformed cells occur either in the bone marrow or the thymus, and they reside in the thymus. The thymic microenvironment, including the epithelial reticular cell network (43, 135), may be essential for the acquisition of T-cell phenotype and the initial proliferation of these cells. The presence of the thymus is not required once these cells become fully autonomous.

The mechanism by which the development of thymic lymphoma is inhibited in partially shielded or bone marrow transplanted irradiated mice (66, 72) might be explained by postulating that either the migration of transformed cells from the bone marrow to the thymus may be overwhelmed by intact marrow cells or the proliferation of transformed cells originating in the thymus might be interfered with and replaced by intact prothymocytes which have migrated from the protected bone marrow.

2. Myeloid leukemogenesis

There are relatively few studies on the mechanism involved in radiation-induced myeloid leukemia in mice compared to thymic lymphoma. However, the development of a quantitative assay method for hematopoietic stem cells and the long-term marrow cell culture system have permitted the analysis of the pathogenesis of myeloid leukemia in connection with stem cell kinetics. Bessho and Hirashima (4) reported that in male RFM mice, overt myeloid leukemia occurred in 24.5% 4–11 months after exposure to a single whole-body X-irradiation of 300 rad, during which the level of colony forming unit in culture (CFU-C) in the marrow was significantly suppressed. The occurrence of the disease ceased as the CFU-C level returned to normal. The potentially neoplastic cells could already be detected as early as 18 days after irradiation, and reached 83.3% of the mice as demonstrated by the transplantation assay method. A significant difference in the incidence of overt leukemia and that of potentially neoplastic cells may imply the intervention of some unknown host defense mechanism. Bessho and Hirashima (4) also observed an increased frequency of myeloid leukemia if X-irradiated mice were given lipopolysaccharide (LPS), which is a potent stimulator for differentiation of CFU-C to granuloid cells through the elevation of the serum colony stimulating factor (CSF). A similar promoting effect of turpentine was previously noted by Upton (124).

Synergism of Radiation and Other Agents

The synergistic action of radiation with other agents is of practical importance. Furth and Boon (20) discussed the synergism between radiation and methylcholanthrene (MC) in the induction of leukemia, and concluded that preirradiation played an important role as a sensitizer of hematopoietic tissue, by which the leukemogenic effect of MC might have been potentiated. The combined treatment of urethane and radiation was also effective in increasing the frequency of leukemia (75). Yokoro et al. (138) demonstrated synergism between radiation and the Gross virus in inducting thymic lymphomas in young adult rats, in which either agent alone was never leukemogenic. The results suggest that radiation acts as a modifier of both the physiologic state of the target cell of the virus and the immunologic responsiveness of the host, whereby an interaction between the target cell and virus, and the proliferation of antigenically altered transformed cells may be promoted. Yokoro et al. (139) also reported the possible role of Gross murine leukemia virus (MuLV) in enhancing the rate of myeloid leukemia induction by X-rays in male RF mice. In contrast to the above mentioned observations, an inhibitory effect of colchicine (76) in the induction of radiogenic leukemia might be attributed to its promotive effect in hematopoietic recovery following radiation injury that is analogous to a similar effect of the normal bone marrow transplantation (72).

Cytogenetic Studies of Radiation-induced Leukemia

Although Kaplan (62) stated that lymphoma cells have the normal diploid complement of 40 chromosomes and there are no chromosome abnormalities during lymphomatous evolution and in established lymphomas of irradiated C57BL mice, others have described various chromosomal aberrations in leukemic and nonleukemic mice following irradiation (17, 57, 104). These discrepancies concerning chromosomal changes in leukemic cells might be due partly to technical difficulties in making preparations in the early days. The improvement of the method for chromosome preparation and the introduction of banding techniques made accurate and detailed observations possible.

Dofuku et al. (14) using the trypsin-Giemsa banding method, first reported the occurrence of trisomies in several chromosomes, especially of No. 15 chromosome in spontaneous thymomas of AKR mice. Subsequent studies revealed that the trisomy of No. 15 chromosome is a nonrandom cytogenetic change and commonly associated with mouse T-cell lymphomas induced by such leukemogenic agents as radiation, chemical carcinogens and leukemogenic viruses (10, 133, 134). The significance of No. 15 trisomy in the pathogenesis of lymphoma is discussed in relation to DNA rearrangements which result in the increased expression of normal cellular genes (79).

In the case of myeloid leukemia in mice, Wald et al. (130) consistently found an extra marker chromosome in bone marrow cells of all the leukemic mice that had been injected previously either with leukemic cells or cell-free centrifugates originally derived from radiation-induced myeloid leukemia in RF mice. They interpreted this together with other findings (56, 109) as evidence that the changes in the chromosome are caused by a virus. Later, Azumi and Sachs (2) described cytogenetic changes that are commonly associated with myeloid leukemia. They found a consistent partial loss of the No. 2 chromosome in myeloid leukemic culture clones established from irradiated SJL/J mice. Their findings were soon confirmed by Japanese workers in radiation-induced myeloid leukemia of C3H/He and RFM mice (40, 41).

The consistent occurrence of these type-specific chromosomal changes in leukemic cells strongly suggests that the changes are associated with the pathogenesis of the respective types of leukemia.

Considerations on the Mechanism of Radiation Leukemogenesis

1. Activation of a latent leukemogenic virus by radiation

Although various factors involved in radiation-induced leukemogenesis in mice have been explored, there is as yet no unified concept of the induction mechanism. As has been pointed out by Kaplan (63) various findings indicate that the mechanism of induction of radiogenic thymic lymphoma is difficult to explain simply as a consequence of the mutagenic effect of radiation on the target cells. The indirect induction mechanism of lymphoma observed in thymectomized X-irradiated thymus-grafted mice could be interpreted as an interaction of nonirradiated lymphoid target cells in the graft and a radiation-activated leukemogenic factor, most likely a virus. In the early 1950s many investigators began to focus their attention on the causative implication of the virus. Interest stemmed from the isolation by Gross of a lymphomagenic virus (passage A virus) from spontaneously developing lymphomas of the AKR mouse (27–29) and Gross was also the first to isolate a lymphomagenic virus (passage X virus) from the lymphoma, originally developed in X-irradiated C3H or C57Br mice. Lieberman and Kaplan (90), motivated by their observation of indirect induction of lymphoma (63) and the successful isolation of a lymphomagenic virus from AKR mice, also attempted cell-free transmission of radiation-induced lymphomas in C57BL/Ka mice to demonstrate the viral nature of the disease. Their effort was not rewarded until they found an efficient way, the intrathymic inoculation of the leukemic cell-free filtrates into suckling mice, resulting in the isolation of a lymphomagenic virus, the Rad LV, which led them to conclude that Rad LV is the direct etiological agent of radiation-induced lymphomas of this mouse strain.

Their interpretation was supported by the electron microscopic demonstration of type-C virus particles in the lymphoreticular tissue of mice shortly after receiving the leukemogenic dose of whole-body X-irradiation (30) and by the demonstration of leukemogenic activity of centrifugates derived from the thymus and bone marrow of X-irradiated nonleukemic mice (34). These findings were strengthened by similar observations of others in the next few years (45, 52, 56, 84). The demonstration that chemically- or hormonally-induced mouse lymphomas (3, 53, 81, 119) were transmissible by cell-free extracts gave additional support to the belief that these leukemogenic agents acted merely as the trigger for the activation of a latent leukemogenic virus already present in the host. However, the origins, mode of transmission, and site or mode of residence of the proposed virus were left unknown.

2.   Oncogene hypothesis and endogenous RNA viruses

In 1969, Huebner and Todaro (48) proposed the hypothesis that genetic information for producing C-type RNA viruses is preserved in every vertebra cell and is vertically transmitted from parent to offspring, and this viral information (virogene including oncogene) plays a key role in transforming a normal cell to a tumor cell. According to the hypothesis, tumorigenic treatment and normal aging trigger the activation of endogenous viral information.

The genetically transmitted endogenous RNA viruses have been subdivided into three classes according to their host range: ecotropic, xenotropic, and amphotropic. The MCF virus, a recombinant virus of ecotropic and xenotropic viruses with amphotropic host range is suspected to be most proximately involved in the development of spontaneous lymphomas (11, 26, 39).

The oncogene hypothesis had considerable impact upon attempts to understand the mechanism of oncogenesis, and its feasibility has been tested in a variety of experimental systems.

Kaplan (64) deduced that at least four different effects of ionizing radiation, acting almost simultaneously in the irradiated host, each contribute to the development of lymphoma following whole-body irradiation: 1) activation of endogenous MuLV replication and mobilization of the virus to the thymus, 2) injury to the thymus followed by a vigorous regeneration, 3) injury to the bone marrow, which in turn interferes with a smooth regeneration of the injured thymus, leading to a state of maturation arrest in which a large number of immature T-lymphocytes become available to interact with the mobilized virus for a sufficient period of time, and 4) immunosuppression caused by both irradiation and MuLV infection, possibly facilitating the proliferation of incipient tumor cells which might have acquired a new antigenic property. An observation of Yokoro et al. (138) that young adult rats which are otherwise resistant to lymphoma induction by the Gross MuLV could be made susceptible to the virus by a sublethal preirradiation of the rats seems to agree with Kaplan's interpretation.

Nagao (105) investigated the appearance of ecotropic MuLV infectivity in various tissues of intact, partial-body shielded or thymectomized female ICR/JCL mice following leukemogenic fractionated X-irradiation to evaluate the correlation between endogenous MuLV infectivity and development of lymphoma in each group. The results indicate that the expression of MuLV may not necessarily be related to the development of lymphoma. Decleve *et al.* (*13*) studied the appearance of Rad LV-associated antigen-positive cells in tissues of C57BL/Ka mice following inoculation of Rad LV which was thought to be the causative agent of radiogenic lymphomas in C57BL/Ka mice. They demonstrated that antigen-positive cells emerged only in the thymus but never in other tissues, the number of positive cells in the thymus increasing gradually during the incubation period, and eventually leading to development of thymic lymphoma. A similar observation was made in W/Fu rats inoculated at birth with the Gross MuLV, in which the exclusive replication of infectious virus in the thymus was associated with the development of thymic lymphomas (*77*).

In contrast to the above, Rad LV-associated antigen-positive cells were rarely found in any tissues of C57BL/Ka mice following leukemogenic X-irradiation (*91*). Ihle *et al.* (*50, 51*) demonstrated in C57BL/6 mice that, although the expression of endogenous ecotropic MuLV was accelerated by leukemogenic irradiation, the peak titer of antibody against gp 71 of the endogenous ecotropic MuLV in irradiated mice was comparable to that in nonirradiated controls, and that the antibody titers were never affected by procedures which lower the leukemia incidence, such as irradiating older mice, low dose irradiation and postirradiation bone marrow transplantation. Furthermore, with rare exceptions, expression of viral antigens was not detected in induced lymphomas. These and other findings (*98*) indicate that the endogenous viruses, at least of ecotropic MuLV, are not playing a major role in mouse radiation-induced leukemogenesis. Moreover, the etiological role of ecotropic MuLV has been negated in chemically-induced leukemogenesis (*106, 107*).

On the other hand, the transient appearance of MuLV gs antigen-positive cells in the bone marrow and thymus of mice several weeks after X-irradiation was interpreted as evidence for the viral involvement even though there was no viral expression in the established lymphoma cells (*33*). Rassart *et al.* (*111*) and Sankar-Mistry *et al.* (*113*) reported that the recombinant B-tropic virus with ecotropic host range is regularly released from cell lines derived from radiogenic lymphomas in C57BL/Ka mice, emphasizing the etiological role of the virus in radiogenic leukemogenesis. However, our observation that there is no evidence of viral implication in cell lines established from radiation- or chemically-induced lymphomas in NFS/N mice may still raise a question to their notion (*136*). There is a report (*92*) suggesting an inhibitory effect of interferon in radiation- and Rad LV-induced leukemogenesis when the leukemogenic stimuli were submaximal. On the contrary, our recent observations that radiation- and chemically-induced mouse leukemogenesis was not affected by treatment with beta-type mouse interferon, while leukemia induction with the Gross MuLV was completely inhibited by the same treatment, also appear to favor the nonviral mechanism of radiation leukemogenesis (Yokoro *et al.* unpublished data).

3. Recently proposed hypothesis

Although MCF virus is the likely etiologic agent in leukemic strains such as AKR and C58 mice, there are no reports suggesting direct involvement of infectious MCF virus in radiation-induced leukemogenesis in low leukemic strains. If so, how are endogenous MuLVs implicated and what is the likely mechanism of radiation-induced leukemogenesis? The following are the hypotheses recently proposed by some investigators.

A) Virus promoter insertion hypothesis

This was first proposed by Hayward *et al.* (*42*) in induction of B-cell lymphoma by

avian leukosis virus which is devoid of viral oncogene (v-onc). They stated that development of lymphoma is due to the activation of a cellular oncogene (c-onc) through the
insertion of a viral promoter sequence adjacent to the c-onc. Repeated virus infection
might be required for the insertion of the promoter at an appropriate location, which
may account for a long latent period of MuLV-induced leukemogenesis as compared to
that of sarcoma induction by murine sarcoma virus (MuSV) that possesses v-onc. Observations in murine virus-induced lymphomas suggest that lymphomagenesis by MuLVs
can result from insertional mutagenesis of cellular oncogenes (*116*).

B) Receptor-mediated leukemogenesis

McGrath and Weissmann (*100, 101*) proposed the receptor-mediated leukemogenesis
hypothesis in which the continued presentation of MuLV env determinant to the cell
surface receptor would act as mitogenic stimuli for the replication of MuLV-induced
lymphoma cells. Ellis *et al.* (*15*) and Tress *et al.* (120) stated that leukemogenesis does
not show a simple dependence on infectious MuLV expression in radiogenic lymphomas,
and that the expression of recombinant env gene product on the lymphoma cells might
play an important role in cell replication. A hypothesis along similar lines has also been
proposed by Lee and Ihle (*88*). Fischinger *et al.* (*16*), analyzing virus-negative radiogenic
lymphoma cells of C57BL/Ka origin, emphasized that binding of nonvirion-associated
permuted gp 70s, which are products of radiation-altered proviral DNA, to cell surface
receptors might act as the signal for autostimulatory blastogenesis, leading to the selective
proliferation of the receptor-bearing T-cells. According to this hypothesis no complete
virus infection or expression of other viral antigens would be required.

C) Oncogene activation

In the past few years, the association of oncogene activation and lymphomagenesis
has been analyzed using both molecular hybridization and gene transfer assays. Activation
of the ras gene family appears rather common in the mouse T-cell lymphomas (*32, 129*).
T lym-1 gene has been isolated from T-cell lymphoma cell lines by molecular cloning
(*83*). In our recent study (*136*), however, there was neither amplification nor rearrange-
ment of env specific genes of MuLV and of cellular oncogenes, such as ras gene family
and myc gene in DNA of NFS cell lines derived from radiation- or chemically-induced
lymphomas. Nevertheless, a molecular approach to lymphomagenesis should be instrumental in elucidating the induction mechanism.

From these hypotheses and observations, there is no doubt that investigations of
viral oncogenesis have contributed much to exploration of the leukemogenic mechanism,
in general, and the author feels that the distinction between viral leukemogenesis and
that induced by other agents is disappearing.

It may also be inferred that infectious endogenous MuLVs as the main cause of
radiation-induced leukemogenesis is probably a rare event, if it occurs at all, but may
rather play a role in certain processes in ways different from those hitherto conceived.
The occasional isolation of leukemogenic viruses from radiation-induced lymphomas may
well represent a rare event.

II. RADIATION-INDUCED MAMMARY CARCINOGENESIS IN RATS

There have been many reports dealing with the mammary carcinogenic effect of
large doses of low LET radiation in rats (*13, 14, 16*), while that of high LET radiation

in low dose ranges has yet to be adequately evaluated. In this review, we present the relevant data in rats recently obtained in our laboratory (27, 28).

Mammary Carcinogenic Effect of Low Dose Fission Neutrons and Other Radiations

1. Induction of mammary tumor (MT) with low doses of fission spectrum neutrons

Studies were undertaken to evaluate the carcinogenic effect of fission neutrons in the low dose range, and the results were compared with those obtained from experiments with 180 kilovolt peak (KvP) X-rays, 14.1 MeV fast neutrons, and 0–0.25 eV thermal neutrons. The rat mammary tumor system has the following advantage as an experimental model for human breast cancer; 1) rat MT is readily induced either by radiation or chemical carcinogens, 2) many rats MTs are hormone dependent or hormone responsive, 3) the majority of rat MTs are of ductal origin as is the case in human, and 4) an increased risk of breast cancer has been observed among women exposed to A-bomb radiation (19–21).

Female W/Fu rats were irradiated at 50 days of age at the Research Reactor Institute, Kyoto University. Irradiation field equivalent to the Hiroshima A-bomb was realized by use of a fission plate (uranium energy converter). Thermal neutrons with an energy of 0.025 eV from the heavy-water thermal neutron facility of KUR (5 mW) (5) at a neutron flux of 3×10^9 n/cm²/sec hit the fission plate; then fast neutrons with average energy of 2.0 MeV and prompt gamma rays were produced by fission reaction of ^{235}U. About 50% of the radiation-initiated rats were further treated with prolactin, the physiological regulatory hormone of mammary tissue, as a promoter to facilitate the detection of the

TABLE I. Induction of MT in Female W/Fu Rats by a Combined Treatment of Fission Radiation and Prolactin

Treatment	Rat with MT / Number in group	Number of MT	Type of MT — Adenoca.	Type of MT — Fibroad.	Latency of MT after irradiation (days)
None	2/24 (8.3%)	3	0	3	597, 843
Prolactin	0/14	—	—	—	—
1.1 rad alone[a]	1/14 (7.1)	1	1	—	304
4.1 rad alone[b]	1/16 (6.3)	1	—	1	205
7.3 rad alone[c]	0/16	—	—	—	—
16.6 rad alone[d]	0/16	—	—	—	—
1.1 rad+prolactin[e]	1/15 (6.7)	1	1	—	237
4.1 rad+prolactin	6/16 (37.5)	6	5	1	191–334
7.3 rad+prolactin	5/15 (33.3)	5	3	2	165–365
16.6 rad+prolactin	9/17 (52.9)	13	7	6	163–365
1.1 rad+prolactin[f]	1/6 (16.7)	1	1	—	502
4.1 rad+prolactin	4/15 (26.7)	6	5	1	463–567
7.3 rad+prolactin	3/15 (20.0)	5	4	1	504–549
16.6 rad+prolactin	4/15 (26.7)	6	5	1	375–526

[a] 0.3 rad fission neutron+0.8 rad gamma rays.
[b] 1.7 rad fission neutron+2.4 rad gamma rays.
[c] 3.3 rad fission neutron+4.0 rad gamma rays.
[d] 8.1 rad fission neutron+8.5 rad gamma rays.
[e] Supply of prolactin was started shortly after irradiation.
[f] Supply of prolactin was started 12 months after irradiation.

carcinogenic effect of radiation. Prolactin was started either a few days or 12 months after irradiation. Experiments were terminated 12–18 months after irradiation.

The incidence, histological type, and latency period of MT in rats of various groups are summarized in Table I. Only 2 of 62 (3.2%) rats receiving 1.0, 4.1, 7.3, or 16.6 rad of fission radiation (composed of both 2.0 MeV fission spectrum neutrons and gamma rays) alone developed MT of benign fibroadenoma type with a long latency period. The induction rate was similar to that of nonirradiated controls. In contrast, 21 of 63 (33.3%) irradiated rats developed MT with a short latency if prolactin was started shortly after irradiation as shown in the middle rows of Table I. The majority of induced MTs were malignant adenocarcinomas. Of 16 rats 6 (37.5%) had MT following exposure to 4.1 rad of fission radiation which contained only 1.7 rad of fission neutron component. The long survival of radiation-initiated potentially malignant cells was apparent when the supply of prolactin to irradiated rats was delayed as late as 12 months after irradiation; 12 of 51 (23.7%) rats developed MT, the frequency of which was comparable to that in rats given prolactin shortly after irradiation (Table I). It is interesting to note that the relative efficacy of MT induction by low dose range of fission radiation appears to be dose in-dependent, the lower dose produced a higher relative risk.

The growth of adenocarcinomas induced by combined treatment of radiation and prolactin was shown to be dependent on both prolactin and ovarian hormones as demon-strated by growth retardation and shrinkage of MT following resection of either grafted prolactin-secreting pituitary tumor or oophorectomy, or both.

2. MT inductivity of ⁶⁰Co gamma rays in low dose range

The mammary carcinogenic effect of gamma rays was tested in order to evaluate the role of gamma rays, which is one component of fission radiation. None of 40 rats exposed to 10 rad of ^{60}Co gamma rays with or without prolactin supply developed MT in an observation period of 12 months, indicating that fission spectrum neutrons played a major role in induction of MT in combination with prolactin.

3. Relative Biological Effectiveness (RBE) of fission spectrum neutrons in induction of rat MT

As stated above, fission spectrum neutrons, especially in the low dose range, were shown to be highly carcinogenic on rat mammary tissue. Therefore, RBE of fission spectrum neutrons for the rat MT inductivity was compared with that of 180 KvP X-rays, 14.1 MeV fast neutrons (27, 28) and 0.025 eV thermal neutrons (unpublished data). We estimated the RBE in such a way as to compare the dose of each radiation type that would produce a MT frequency which was 40% of the incidence in irradiated rats treated with prolactin. The doses of each radiation type which induced 40% incidence were: 50 rad of X-rays, 35.4 rad of fast neutrons, 7.4 rad of thermal neutrons, and 2.8 rad

TABLE II. Differences in MT Inductivity of Various Radiations in Female W/Fu Rats as Detected by the Promotive Effect of Prolactin

	Fission neutrons (2.0 MeV)	Thermal neutrons (0.025 eV)	Fast neutrons (14.1 MeV)	X-rays (180 kVp)
Dose (rad) giving 40% of MT incidence	2.8	7.4	35.4	50
RBE for MT inductivity	17.8	6.7	1.4	1

of fission neutrons, respectively. Since gamma rays play a minor role in rat mammary carcinogenesis as described in the previous section, the gamma ray component was arbitrarily ignored for the latter two radiation types. As shown in Table II, it is clear that the efficiency of 2.0 MeV fission spectrum neutrons is much higher than those of others; RBE of fission spectrum neutrons is 17.8 against 180 KvP X-rays.

DISCUSSION

We have demonstrated that the mammary carcinogenic effect of apparently sub-carcinogenic doses of fission neutrons could be promoted by elevating prolactin levels in irradiated rats.

The determining role of prolactin in the induction and maintenance of the growth of murine mammary carcinogenesis has been well documented (3, 6, 9, 18, 24–26), from which the importance of prolactin in human breast carcinogenesis is easily conceived. However, the findings have been conflicting with respect to the serum prolactin levels of breast cancer patients (1, 4, 8, 12, 17). Taking a general view of the implication of prolactin in normal and transformed mammary epithelial cells in both rodents and humans, it is assumed that the elevation of prolactin level to a certain extent, with other favorable host factors, is a prerequisite for the induction and further development of MT regardless of the species.

It has been well documented that the relative risk of MT has been increasing among women who were exposed to A-bomb radiation, and the effect is dose dependent (19–21). The long latency of MT development among survivors suggests that long-surviving radiation-initiated dormant cancer cells may exist in the mammary tissue and that those cancer cells begin to proliferate in response to the change in certain host and other environmental factors. This supposition is supported by our data in rats (27, 28).

Vogel (22), Vogel and Zaldiver (23), and Shellabarger et al. (15) reported an extremely high RBE of 0.43 MeV or 1.2 MeV fission neutrons as compared with 250 KvP X-rays for the induction of rat MT. Montour et al. (7) and Clifton et al. (2) also stressed the high efficiency of neutrons in different experimental systems. Furthermore, all these authors emphasized that the high RBE of neutrons was more prominent in the low dose range and that the RBE of neutrons decreases as dose increases.

CLOSING REMARKS

Almost half a century has passed since experimental study, mainly of mice, was introduced as a model system for studying the etiology, pathophysiology, and treatment of human leukemia. At present, a counterpart for almost every form of human leukemia can be induced in rodents by the skillful use of various leukemogens including ionizing radiation. Furthermore, recent advances in immunology, genetics, tumor virology, and molecular biology have been incorporated into leukemia research, resulting in rapid progress, especially with respect to T-cell lymphoma and lymphoid leukemia.

Continued efforts along these lines will enable us to arrive at a unified concept of radiation-induced leukemogenesis in the not too distant future.

The experimental findings described in this review, particularly those related to radiation-induced mammary carcinogenesis, may have some relevance to the recent investigations for reassessment of gamma ray and neutron radiation dose produced by the A-bombs in Hiroshima and Nagasaki (*10, 11*). Although our evidence shows that neutrons can be effective in animal carcinogenesis, there seems no human population available for comparison, since it is now known that the neutron dose in Hiroshima and Nagasaki was so small that the effects cannot be adequately assessed.

Acknowledgment

All of our studies described in this review were performed under the support of a Grant-in-Aid for Cancer Research from the Ministry of Education, Science and Culture, Japan.

REFERENCES

I. Radiation-Induced Leukemogenesis in Mice

1. A review of thirty years study of Hiroshima and Nagasaki atomic bomb survivors, *J. Radiat. Res.*, **16** (Suppl.), 1–164 (1975).

2. Azumi, J. and Sachs, L. Chromosome mapping of the genes that control differentiation and malignancy in myeloid leukemia cells. *Proc. Natl. Acad. Sci. U.S.A.*, **74**, 253–257 (1977).

3. Ball, J. K. and McCarter, J. A. Repeated demonstration of a mouse leukemia virus after treatment with chemical carcinogens. *J. Natl. Cancer Inst.*, **46**, 751–762 (1971).

4. Bessho, M. and Hirashima, K. Experimental studies on the mechanism of leukemogenesis following the hemopoietic stem cell kinetics. *Acta Haematol. Jpn.*, **45**, 1296–1306 (1982).

5. Boniver, J., Decleve, A., Lieberman, M., Honsik, C., Travis, M., and Kaplan, H. S. Marrow-thymus interactions during radiation leukemogenesis in C57BL/Ka mice. *Cancer Res.*, **41**, 390–392 (1981).

6. Boniver, J., Simar, L. J., Courtoy, R., and Betz, E. H. Quantitative analysis of thymus lymphoid cells during murine radioleukemogenesis. *Cancer Res.*, **38**, 52–58 (1978).

7. Brues, A. M., Aacher, G. A., Finkel, M. P., and Lisco, H. Comparative carcinogenic effects by X-radiation and P^{32}. *Cancer Res.*, **9**, 545 (1949).

8. Burrows, H. and Cook, J. W. Spindle-cell tumours and leucaemia in mice after injection with a water soluble compound of 1:2:5:6-dibenzanthracene. *Am J. Cancer*, **27**, 267–278 (1936).

9. Carnes, W. H., Kaplan, H. S., Brown, M. B., and Hirsch, B. B. Indirect induction of lymphomas in irradiated mice. III. Role of the thymic graft. *Cancer Res.*, **16**, 429–433 (1956).

10. Chan, F.P.H., Ball, J. K., and Sergovich, F. R. Trisomy #15 in murine thymomas induced by chemical carcinogens, x-irradiation, and an endogenous murine leukemia virus. *J. Natl. Cancer Inst.*, **62**, 605–610 (1979).

11. Cloyd, M. W., Hartley, J. W., and Rowe, W. P. Lymphomagenicity of recombinant mink cell focus-inducing murine leukemia viruses. *J. Exp. Med.*, **151**, 542–552 (1980).

12. Congdon, C. C., Uphoff, D., and Lorenz, E. Modification of acute irradiation injury in mice and guinea pigs by injection of bone marrow: A histopathologic study. *J. Natl. Cancer Inst.*, **13**, 73–107 (1952).

13. Decleve, A., Sato, C., Lieberman, M., and Kaplan, H. S. Selective thymic localization of murine leukemia virus-related antigens in C57BL/Ka mice after inoculation with Radiation Leukemia Virus. *Proc. Natl. Acad. Sci. U.S.A.*, **71**, 3124–3128 (1974).

14. Dofuku, R., Biedler, J. L., Spengler, B. A., and Old, L. J. Trisomy of chromosome 15 in spontaneous leukemias of AKR mice. *Proc. Natl. Acad. Sci. U.S.A.*, **72**, 1515–1517 (1975).

15. Ellis, R. W., Stockert, E., and Fleissner, E. Association of endogenous retroviruses with radiation-induced leukemias of BALB/c mice. *J. Virol.*, **33**, 652–660 (1980).

16. Fischinger, P. J., Thiel, H. J., Lieberman, M., Kaplan, H. S., Dunlop, N. M. and Robey, W. G. Presence of a novel recombinant murine leukemia virus-like glycoprotein on the surface of virus-negative C57BL lymphoma cells. *Cancer Res.*, **42**, 4650–4657 (1982).

17. Ford, C. E., Hamerton, J. L., and Mole, R. H. Chromosomal changes in primary and transplanted reticular neoplasms of the mouse. *J. Cell Comp. Physiol.*, **1** (Suppl.), 235–269 (1958).

18. Fry, R.J.M., Experimental radiation carcinogenesis: What have we learned? *Radiat. Res.*, **87**, 224–239 (1981).

19. Furth, J. The creation of the AKR strain, whose DNA contains the genome of a leukemia virus. *In* "Origins of Inbred Mice," ed. H. C. Morse III, pp. 69–97 (1978). Academic Press, New York.

20. Furth, J. and Boon, M. C. Enhancement of leukemogenic action of methylcholanthrene by preirradiation with x-rays. *Science*, **98**, 133–139 (1943).

21. Furth, J. and Boon, M. C. The time and site of origin of the leukemic cells. AAAS Research Conference on Cancer, pp. 129–138 (1944).

22. Furth, J. and Furth, O. B. Neoplastic disease produced in mice by general irradiation with x-rays. 1. Incidence and type of neoplasms. *Am. J. Cancer*, **28**, 54–65 (1936).

23. Furth, J. and Furth, O. B. Monocytic leukemia and other neoplastic diseases occurring in mice following intrasplenic injection of 1:2-benzpyrene. *Am. J. Cancer*, **34**, 169–183 (1938).

24. Furth, J. and Lorenz, E. Carcinogenesis by ionizing radiation. *In* "Radiation Biology," ed. A. Hollander, pp. 1145–1201 (1954). McGraw Hill, New York.

25. Furth, J., Seibold, H. R., and Rathbone, R. R. Experimental studies on lymphomatosis of mice. *Am. J. Cancer*, **19**, 521–604 (1933).

26. Green, N., Hiai, H., Elder, J. H., Schwartz, R. S., Khiroya, R. H., Thomas, C. Y., Tsichles, P. N., and Coffin, J. M. Expression of leukemogenic recombinant viruses associated with a recessive gene in HRS/J mice. *J. Exp. Med.*, **152**, 249–264 (1980).

27. Gross, L. "Spontaneous" leukemia developing in C3H mice following inoculation, in infancy, with Ak-leukemic extracts, or Ak-embryos. *Proc. Soc. Exp. Biol. Med.*, **76**, 27–32 (1951).

28. Gross, L. Development and serial cell-free passage of a highly potent strain of mouse leukemia virus. *Proc. Soc. Exp. Biol. Med.*, **94**, 767–771 (1957).

29. Gross, L. Serial cell-free passage of a radiation-activated mouse leukemia agent. *Proc. Soc. Exp. Biol. Med.*, **100**, 102–105 (1959).

30. Gross, L. and Feldman, G. G. Electron microscopic studies of radiation-induced leukemia in mice: virus release following total-body x-ray irradiation. *Cancer Res.*, **28**, 1677–1685 (1968).

31. Gross, L., Roswit, B., Mada, E. R., Dreyfuss, Y., and Moore, L. A. Studies on radiation-induced leukemia in mice. *Cancer Res.*, **19**, 316–320 (1959).

32. Guerrero, I., Calzada, P., Mayer, A., and Pellicer, A. A molecular approach to leukemogenesis: Mouse lymphomas contain an activated c-ras oncogene. *Proc. Natl. Acad. Sci. U.S.A.*, **81**, 202–205 (1984).

33. Haas, M. Transient virus expression during murine leukemia induction by x-irradiation. *J. Natl. Cancer Inst.*, **58**, 251–257 (1977).

34. Haran-Ghera, N. Leukemogenic activity of centrifugates from irradiated mouse thymus and bone marrow. *Int. J. Cancer*, **1**, 81–87 (1966).

35. Haran-Ghera, N. Pathways in murine radiation leukemogenesis-coleukemogenesis. *In* "Biology of Radiation Carcinogenesis," ed. J. Yuhas, R. Tennant, and J. Regen, pp. 245–260 (1976). Raven Press, New York.

36. Haran-Ghera, N. Target cells involved in radiation leukemia virus leukemogenesis. *In*

"International Symposium on Radiation Induced Leukemogenesis and Related Viruses, INSERM Symp. No. 4," ed. J. F. Duplan, pp. 79–89 (1977). Elsevier/North Holland Biomedical Press, Amsterdam.

37. Haran-Ghera, N. and Kaplan, H. S. Significance of thymus and marrow injury in urethan leukemogenesis. *Cancer Res.*, **24**, 1926–1931 (1964).

38. Haran-Ghera, N. and Peled, A. The mechanism of radiation action in leukemogenesis. IV. Immune impairment as a coleukemogenic factor. *Isr. J. Med. Sci.*, **4**, 1181–1187 (1968).

39. Hartley, J. W., Wolford, N. K., Old, L. J., and Rowe, W. P. A new class of murine leukemia virus associated with development of spontaneous lymphomas. *Proc. Natl. Acad. Sci. U.S.A.*, **74**, 789–792 (1977).

40. Hayata, I., Ishihara, T., Hirashima, K., Sado, T., and Yamagiwa, J. Partial deletion of chromosome #2 in myelocytic leukemias of irradiated C3H/He and RFM mice. *J. Natl. Cancer Inst.*, **63**, 843–848 (1979).

41. Hayata, I., Seki, M., Yoshida, K., Hirashima, K., Sado, T., Yamagiwa, J., and Ishihara, T. Chromosomal aberrations observed in 52 mouse myeloid leukemias. *Cancer Res.*, **43**, 367–373 (1983).

42. Hayward, W. S., Neel, B. G., and Astrin, S. M. Activation of a cellular onc gene by promoter insertion in ALV-induced lymphoid leukosis. *Nature*, **290**, 475–480 (1981).

43. Hiai, N., Nishi, Y., Miyazawa, T., Matsudaira, Y., and Nishizuka, Y. Mouse lymphoid leukemias: Symbiotic complexes of neoplastic lymphocytes and their microenvironments. *J. Natl. Cancer Inst.*, **66**, 713–722 (1981).

44. Hiraki, K., Irino, S., and Sota, S. Studies on cytogenesis of RF mouse leukemia induced by X-ray irradiation. Proc. 8th Congr. Europ. Soc. Hematol., p. 347 (1962).

45. Hiraki, K., Irino, S., Sota, S., and Ikejiri, K. Leukemogenic activity of cell-free filtrates of radiation-induced leukemia of RF mice. *J. Radiat. Res.*, **5**, 1–11 (1964).

46. Hormberg, E.A.D., De Pasqualini, C. D., Arini, E., Pavlovsky, A., and Rabasa, S. L. Leukemogenic effect of radioactive phosphorous in adult and fetally exposed BALB mice. *Cancer Res.*, **24**, 1745–1748 (1964).

47. Hormberg, E.A.D., Vasquez, C., De Pasqualini, C. D., Pavlovsky, A., and Rabasa, S. L. A cellular passage of ^{32}P-induced leukemia; an electron microscopic study. *Cancer Res.*, **27**, 198–204 (1967).

48. Huebner, R. J. and Todaro, G. J. Oncogenes of RNA tumor viruses as determinants of cancer. *Proc. Natl. Acad. Sci. U.S.A.*, **64**, 1087–1094 (1969).

49. Hueper, W. C. Leukemoid and leukemic conditions in white mice with spontaneous mammary carcinoma. *Folia Haematol.*, **52**, 167–178 (1934).

50. Ihle, J. N., Joseph, D. R., and Pazmino, N. H. Radiation leukemia in C57BL/6 mice. II. Lack of ecotropic virus expression in the majority of lymphomas. *J. Exp. Med.*, **144**, 1406–1423 (1976).

51. Ihle, J. N., McEwan, R., and Bengali, K. Radiation leukemia in C57BL/6 mice. 1. Lack of serological evidence for the role of endogenous ecotropic viruses in pathogenesis. *J. Exp. Med.*, **144**, 1391–1405 (1976).

52. Ilbery, P.L.T. and Winn, S. M. Indirect transfer of radiogenic lymphoma. *Aust. J. Exp. Biol. Med. Sci.*, **42**, 133–148 (1964).

53. Irino, S., Ota, Z., Sezaki, T., Suzaki, M., and Hiraki, K. Cell-free transmission of 20-methylcholanthrene-induced RF mouse leukemia and electron microscopic demonstration of virus particles in its leukemic tissue. *Gann*, **54**, 225–237 (1963).

54. Ito, T., Nagao, K., Kawamura, Y., and Yokoro, K. Studies on the leukemogenic and immunologic effects of radiostrontium (^{90}Sr) and X-rays in mice. *In* "Proc. 14th Annual Hanford Biology Symp. of Radiation and the Lymphatic System, ERDA Symp. Series 37," pp. 209–217 (1976). National Technical Information Service, US Dept. of Commerce, Springfield.

55. Ito, T., Yokoro, K., Ito, A., and Nishihara, E. A comparative study of the leukemogenic effects of strontium-90 and x-rays in mice. *Proc. Soc. Exp. Biol. Med.*, **130**, 345–350 (1969).

56. Jenkins, V. K. and Upton, A. C. Cell-free transmission of radiogenic myeloid leukemia in the mouse. *Cancer Res.*, **23**, 1748–1755 (1963).

57. Joneja, M. G. and Stich, H. F. Chromosomes of tumor cells. IV. Cell population changes in thymus, spleen, and bone marrow during X-ray-induced leukemogenesis in C57BL/6J mice. *J. Natl. Cancer Inst.*, **35**, 421–434 (1965).

58. Kaplan, H. S. Observations on radiation-induced lymphoid tumors of mice. *Cancer Res.*, **7**, 141–147 (1947).

59. Kaplan, H. S. Comparative susceptibility of the lymphoid tissues of strain C57 Black mice to the induction of lymphoid tumors by irradiation. *J. Natl. Cancer Inst.*, **8**, 191–197 (1948).

60. Kaplan, H. S. Preliminary studies on the effectiveness of local irradiation in the induction of lymphoid tumors in mice. *J. Natl. Cancer Inst.*, **10**, 267–270 (1949).

61. Kaplan, H. S. Influence of thymectomy, splenectomy, and gonadectomy on incidence of radiation-induced lymphoid tumors in strain C57 Black mice. *J. Natl. Cancer Inst.*, **11**, 83–90 (1950).

62. Kaplan, H. S. The nature of the neoplastic transformation in lymphoid tumour induction. *In* "Ciba Foundation Symposium on Carcinogenesis, Mechanism of Action," pp. 233–244 (1959). Little Brown, Boston.

63. Kaplan, H. S. On the natural history of the murine leukemias: Presidential address. *Cancer Res.*, **27**, 1325–1340 (1967).

64. Kaplan, H. S. Leukemia and lymphoma in experimental and domestic animals. *Ser. Haemat.*, **VII**, (2), 94–163 (1974).

65. Kaplan, H. S. Interaction between radiation and viruses in the induction of murine thymic lymphomas and lymphatic leukemias. *In* "International Symposium on Radiation-induced Leukemogenesis and Related Viruses, INSERM Symp. No. 4," ed. J. F. Duplan, pp. 1–18 (1977). Elsevier/North Holland Biomedical Press, Amsterdam.

66. Kaplan, H. S. and Brown, M. B. Protection against radiation-induced lymphoma development by shielding and partial-body irradiation of mice. *Cancer Res.*, **12**, 441–444 (1952).

67. Kaplan, H. S. and Brown, M. B. Testosterone prevention of post-irradiation lymphomas in C57 Black mice. *Cancer Res.*, **12**, 445–447 (1952).

68. Kaplan, H. S. and Brown, M. B. Mortality of mice after total-body irradiation as influenced by alterations in total dose fractionation, and periodicity of treatment. *J. Natl. Cancer Inst.*, **12**, 765–775 (1952).

69. Kaplan, H. S. and Brown, M. B. A quantitative dose-response study of lymphoid-tumor development in irradiated C57 Black mice. *J. Natl. Cancer Inst.*, **13**, 185–208 (1952).

70. Kaplan, H. S., Brown, M. B., Hirsch, B. B., and Carnes, W. H. Indirect induction of lymphomas in irradiated mice. II. Factor of irradiation of the host. *Cancer Res.*, **16**, 426–428 (1956).

71. Kaplan, H. S., Brown, M. B., and Paull, J. Influence of post-irradiation thymectomy and of thymic implants on lymphoid tumor incidence in C57BL mice. *Cancer Res.*, **13**, 677–680 (1953).

72. Kaplan, H. S., Brown, M. B., and Paull, J. Influence of bone marrow injections on involution and neoplasia of mouse thymus after systemic irradiation. *J. Natl. Cancer. Inst.*, **14**, 303–316 (1953).

73. Kaplan, H. S., Carnes, W. H., Brown, M. B., and Hirsch, B. B. Indirect induction of lymphomas in irradiated mice. 1. Tumor incidence and morphology in mice bearing non-irradiated thymic grafts. *Cancer Res.*, **16**, 422–425 (1956).

74. Kaplan, H. S., Hirsch, B. B., and Brown, M. B. Indirect induction of lymphomas in irradiated mice. IV. Genetic evidence of the origin of the tumor cells from the thymic grafts. *Cancer Res.*, **16**, 434–436 (1956).

75. Kawamoto, S., Ida, N., Kirschbaum, A., and Taylor, H. G. Urethane and leukemogenesis in mice. *Cancer Res.*, **18**, 725–729 (1958).

76. Kawamoto, S., Kirschbaum, A., Trentin, J. J., and Taylor, H. G. Influence of colchicine on leukemogenic effect of X-ray, estrogen, methylcholanthrene, and urethane in mice. *Cancer Res.*, **21**, 309–313 (1961).

77. Kawamura, Y. Type-C RNA viruses and leukemogenesis: Association of Gross strain of murine leukemia virus infection and leukemogenesis in rats. *J. Natl. Cancer Inst.*, **56**, 927–930 (1976).

78. Kirschbaum, A., Shapiro, J. R., and Mixer, H. W. Synergistic action of estrogenic hormone and X-rays in inducing thymic lymphosarcoma of mice. *Proc. Soc. Exp. Biol. Med.*, **72**, 632–634 (1949).

79. Klein, G. The role of gene dosage and genetic transpositions in carcinogenesis. *Nature*, **294**, 313–318 (1981).

80. Krebs, G., Rask-Nielsen, H. C., and Wagner, A. The origin of lymphosarcomatosis and its relation to other forms of leucosis in white mice. *Acta Radiol.*, **10** (Suppl.), 1–53 (1930).

81. Kunii, A., Takemoto, H., and Furth, J. Leukemogenic filtrable agent from estrogen-induced thymic lymphoma in RF mice. *Proc. Soc. Exp. Biol. Med.*, **119**, 1211–1215 (1965).

82. Lacassagne, A. Sarcomas lymphoides apparus chez des souris longuement traitees par des hormones oestrogenes. *Compt. Rend. Soc. Biol.*, **126**, 193–195 (1937).

83. Lane, M., Sainten, A., Doherty, K. M., and Cooper, G. M. Isolation and characterization of a stage-specific transforming gene, T lym-1, from T-cell lymphomas. *Proc. Natl. Acad. Sci. U.S.A.*, **81**, 2227–2231 (1984).

84. Latarjet, R. and Duplan, J. F. Experiment and discussion on leukemogenesis by cell-free extracts of radiation-induced leukemia in mice. *Int. J. Radiat. Biol.*, **5**, 339–344 (1962).

85. Law, L. W. and Miller, J. H. Observations on the effect of thymectomy on spontaneous leukemias in mice of high leukemia strains RIL and C58. *J. Natl. Cancer Inst.*, **11**, 253–262 (1950).

86. Law, L. W. and Miller, J. H. The influence of thymectomy on the incidence of carcinogen-induced leukemia in strain DBA mice. *J. Natl. Cancer Inst.*, **11**, 425–437 (1950).

87. Law, L. W. and Potter, M. The behavior in transplant of lymphocytic neoplasms arising from parental thymic grafts in irradiated, thymectomized hybrid mice. *Proc. Natl. Acad. Sci. U.S.A.*, **42**, 160–167 (1956).

88. Lee, J. C. and Ihle, J. N. Mechanisms of C-type viral leukemogenesis. I. Correlation of *in vitro* lymphocyte blastogenesis to viremina and leukemia. *J. Immunol.*, **123**, 2351–2358 (1979).

89. Levinthal, J. D., Buffett, R. F., and Furth, J. Prevention of viral leukemia of mice by thymectomy. *Proc. Soc. Exp. Biol. Med.*, **100**, 610–614 (1959).

90. Lieberman, M. and Kaplan, H. S. Leukemogenic activity of filtrates from radiation-induced lymphoid tumors of mice. *Science*, **130**, 387–388 (1959).

91. Lieberman, M., Kaplan, H. S., and Decleve, A. Anomalous viral expression in radiogenic lymphomas of C57BL/Ka mice. *In* "Biology of Radiation Carcinogenesis," ed. J. M. Yuhas, R. W. Tennant, and J. D. Regen, pp. 237–244 (1976). Raven Press, New York.

92. Lieberman, M., Merigan, T. C., and Kaplan, H. S. Inhibition of radiogenic lymphoma development in mice by interferon. *Proc. Soc. Exp. Biol. Med.*, **138**, 575–578 (1971).

93. Lorenz, E. Effects of long-continued total-body gamma irradiation on mice, guinea pigs, and rabbits. III. Effects on life span, weight, blood picture, and carcinogenesis and the role of intensity of radiation. *In* "National Nuclear Energy Series, IV-22B," ed. R. E. Zirkle, pp. 24–148 (1954). McGraw Hill, New York.

94. Lorenz, E. and Congdon, C. C. Modification of lethal irradiation injury in mice by injection of homologous or heterologous bone. *J. Natl. Cancer Inst.*, **14**, 955–965 (1954).

95. Lorenz, E., Congdon, C. C., and Uphoff, D. Prevention of irradiation induced lymphoid

tumors in C57BL mice by spleen protection. *J. Natl. Cancer Inst.*, **14**, 291–297 (1953).

96. Loutit, J. F. Protection against ionizing radiation. The "recovery factor" in spleen and bone marrow. *J. Nucl. Energy*, **1**, 87–91 (1954).
97. March, H. C. Leukemia in radiologists. *Radiology*, **43**, 275–278 (1944).
98. Mayer, A. and Dorsch-Häsler, K. Endogenous MuLV infection does not contribute to onset of radiation- or carcinogen-induced murine thymoma. *Nature*, **295**, 253–255 (1982).
99. McEndy, D. P., Boon, M. C., and Furth, J. On the role of thymus, spleen, and gonads in the development of leukemia in a high-leukemia stock of mice. *Cancer Res.*, **4**, 377–383 (1944).
100. McGrath, M. S., Pillemer, E., and Weissman, I. L. Murine leukemogenesis: monoclonal antibodies to T-cell determinants arrest T-lymphoma cell proliferation. *Nature*, **285**, 259–261 (1980).
101. McGrath, M. S. and Weissman, I. L. AKR leukemogenesis; identification and biological significance of thymic lymphoma receptors for KAK retroviruses. *Cell*, **17**, 65–75 (1979).
102. Miller, J.F.A.P. Role of the thymus in virus-induced leukemia. *In* "Ciba Found. Symp. on Tumour Viruses of Murine Origin," ed. G.E.W. Wolstenholme and M. O'Connor, pp. 262–279 (1962). J. & A. Churchill, London.
103. Muto, M., Sado, T., Hayata, I., Kamisaku, H., Nagasawa, F., and Kubo, E. Reconfirmation of indirect induction of radiogenic lymphomas using thymectomized, irradiated B10 mice grafted with neonatal thymuses from Thy 1 congenic donors. *Cancer Res.*, **43**, 3822–3827 (1983).
104. Nadler, C. F. Chromosomal patterns of irradiated leukemic and non-leukemic C57BL/6J mice. *J. Natl. Cancer Inst.*, **30**, 923–931 (1963).
105. Nagao, K. Type-C RNA virus and leukemogenesis: lack of correlation between expression of endogenous, ecotropic murine leukemia virus and radiation leukemogenesis in mice. *Hiroshima J. Med. Sci.*, **26**, 177–188 (1977).
106. Nexo, B. A. and Ulrich, K. Activation of C-type virus during chemically induced leukemogenesis in mice. *Cancer Res.*, **38**, 729–735 (1978).
107. Odaka, T. Strain-dependent expression of endogenous mouse-tropic viruses in chemically induced murine leukemias. *Int. J. Cancer*, **16**, 622–628 (1975).
108. Parkinson, D. R., Brightman, R. P., and Waksal, S. D. Altered natural killer cell biology in C57BL/6 mice after leukemogenic split-dose irradiation. *J. Immunol.*, **126**, 1460–1464 (1981).
109. Parsons, D. F., Upton, A. C., Bender, M. A., Jenkins, V. K., Nelson, E. S., and Johnson, R. R. Electron microscopic observations on primary and serially passaged radiation-induced myeloid leukemias of the RF mice. *Cancer Res.*, **22**, 728–736 (1962).
110. Rappaport, H. and Baroni, C. A study of the pathogenesis of malignant lymphoma induced in the Swiss mouse by 7, 12-dimethylbenz(a)anthracene injected at birth. *Cancer Res.*, **22**, 1067–1074 (1962).
111. Rassart, E., Sankar-Mistry, P., Lemay, G., Des Grosseillers, L., and Jolicoeur, P. New class of leukemogenic ecotropic recombinant murine leukemia virus isolated from radiation-induced thymomas of C57BL/6 mice. *J. Virol.*, **45**, 565–575 (1983).
112. Sado, T. (personal communication from National Institute of Radiological Sciences, Chiba, Japan) (1983).
113. Sankar-Mistry, P. and Jolicoeur, P. Frequent isolation of ecotropic murine leukemia virus after x-ray irradiation of C57BL/6 mice and establishment of producer lymphoid cell lines from radiation-induced lymphomas. *J. Virol.*, **35**, 270–275 (1980).
114. Sasaki, S. and Kasuga, T. Life-shortening and carcinogenesis in mice irradiated neonatally with x rays. *Radiat. Res.*, **88**, 313–325 (1981).
115. Siegler, R., Harrell, W., and Rich, M. A. Pathogenesis of radiation-induced thymic lymphoma in mice. *J. Natl. Cancer Inst.*, **37**, 105–121 (1966).

116. Steffen, D. Proviruses are adjacent to c-myc in some murine leukemia virus-induced lymphomas. *Proc. Natl. Acad. Sci. U.S.A.*, **81**, 2097–2101 (1984).

117. Takizawa, S., Ito, A., Kawase, A., Yamasaki, T., Nishihara, H., and Yokoro, K. Induction of leukemia in mice with radioactive phosphorus (^{32}P) and its modification by thymectomy and splenectomy. *J. Kyushu Hematol. Soc.*, **18**, 1–7 (1968) (in Japanese with English abstr.)

118. Toch, P., Hirsch, B. B., Brown, M. B., Nagareda, C. S., and Kaplan, H. S. Lymphoid tumor incidence in mice treated with estrogen and X-radiation. *Cancer Res.*, **16**, 890–893 (1956).

119. Toth, B. Development of malignant lymphomas by cell-free filtrates prepared from a chemically induced mouse lymphoma. *Proc. Soc. Exp. Biol. Med.*, **112**, 873–875 (1963).

120. Tress, E., Pierotti, M., De Leo, A. B., O'Donnell, P. V., and Fleissner, E. Endogenous murine leukemia virus-encoded proteins in radiation leukemias of BALB/c mice. *Virology*, **117**, 207–218 (1982).

121. Ullrich, R. L., Jernigan, M. C., Cosgrove, G. E., Satterfield, L. C., Bowles, N. D., and Storer, J. B. The influence of dose and dose rate on the induction of neoplastic disease in RFM mice after neutron irradiation. *Radiat. Res.*, **68**, 115–131 (1976).

122. Ullrich, R. L. and Storer, J. B. Influence of gamma irradiation on the development of neoplastic disease in mice. 1. Reticular tissue tumors. *Radiat. Res.*, **80**, 303–316 (1979).

123. Ulrich, H. The incidence of leukemia in radiologists. *New Engl. J. Med.*, **234**, 45–46 (1946).

124. Upton, A. C. Studies on the mechanism of leukemogenesis by ionizing radiation. *In* "Carcinogenesis, Mechanism of Action," A Ciba Found. Symp., ed. G.E.W. Wolstenholme, pp. 249–268 (1959). Little Brown, Boston.

125. Upton, A. C. Experimental radiation-induced leukemia. *In* "International Symposium on Radiation-induced Leukemogenesis and Related Viruses. INSERM Symp. No. 4," ed. J. F. Duplan, pp. 37–50 (1977). Elsevier/North-Holland, Amsterdam.

126. Upton, A. C., Randolph, M. L., and Conklin, J. W. Late effects of fast neutrons and gamma rays in mice as influenced by the dose rate of irradiation: Induction of neoplasia. *Radiat. Res.*, **41**, 467–491 (1970).

127. Upton, A. C., Wolff, F. F., Furth, J., and Kimball, A. W. A comparison of the induction of myeloid and lymphoid leukemias in X-radiated RF mice. *Cancer Res.*, **18**, 842–848 (1958).

128. Van Jagic, N., Schwartz, G., and Siebenrock, L. V. Blutbefunde bein Röntgenologen. *Berliner Klin. Wochenschr.*, **48**, 1220–1222 (1911).

129. Vousden, K. H. and Marshall, C. J. Three different activated ras genes in mouse tumours; evidence for oncogene activation during progression of a mouse lymphoma. *EMBO J.*, **3**, 913–917 (1984).

130. Wald, N., Upton, A. C., Jenkins, V. K., and Borges, W. H. Radiation-induced mouse leukemia; consistent occurrence of an extra and a marker chromosome. *Science*, **143**, 810–813 (1964).

131. Warner, J. F. and Dennert, G. Effects of a cloned cell line with NK activity on bone marrow transplants, tumour development and metastasis *in vivo*. *Nature*, **300**, 31–34 (1982).

132. Wasi, P. and Block, M. The histopathologic study of the development of the irradiation-induced leukemia in C57BL mice and its inhibition by testosterone. *Cancer Res.*, **21**, 463–473 (1961).

133. Wiener, F., Ohno, S., Spira, J., Haran-Ghera, N., and Klein, G. Chromosome changes (Trisomies 15 and 17) associated with tumor progression in leukemia induced by radiation leukemia virus. *J. Natl. Cancer Inst.*, **61**, 227–237 (1978).

134. Wiener, F., Spira, J., Ohno, S., Haran-Ghera, N., and Klein, G. Chromosome changes

(Trisomy 15) in murine T-cell leukemia induced by 7, 12-dimethylbenz(a)anthracene (DMBA). *Int. J. Cancer*, **22**, 447–453 (1978).

135. Yanagihara, K., Kajitani, T., Kamiya, K., and Yokoro, K. *In vitro* studies on the mechanism of leukemogenesis. 1. Establishment and characterization of cell lines derived from the thymic epithelial reticulum cell of the mouse. *Leukemia Res.*, **5**, 321–329 (1981).

136. Yanagihara, K., Seyama, T., and Yokoro, K. Establishment of virus-negative cell lines derived from radiation- or chemically-induced T-cell lymphomas in NFS/N mice, and generation of oncogenic virus from these cell lines following infection of a non-oncogenic ecotropic virus. *In* "RNA Tumor Viruses, Oncogenes, Human Cancer and Aids: On the Frontiers of Understanding," ed. P. Furmanski, J. C. Hager, and M. A. Rich, pp. 372–381 (1985). Martinus Nijhoff, Boston.

137. Yokoro, K., Imamura, N., Kajihara, H., Nakano, M., and Takizawa, S. Association of virus in radiation and chemical leukemogenesis in rats and mice. *In* "Unifying Concepts of Leukemia," ed. R. M. Dutcher and L. Chieco-Bianchi, pp. 603–616 (1973). Karger, Basel.

138. Yokoro, K., Ito, T., Imamura, N., Kawase, A., and Yamasaki, T. Synergistic action of radiation and virus in induction of leukemia in rats. *Cancer Res.*, **29**, 1973–1976 (1969).

139. Yokoro, K., Takemoto, H., and Kunii, A. Role of lymphoma virus in induction of myeloid leukemia by X-rays. *Ann. N.Y. Acad. Sci.*, **114** (part 1), 203–212 (1964).

II. Radiation-Induced Mammary Carcinogenesis in Rats

1. Boyns, A. R., Cole, E. N., and Griffiths, K. Plasma prolactin in breast cancer. *Eur. J. Cancer*, **9**, 99–102 (1973).

2. Clifton, K. H., Douple, E. B., and Sridharan, B. N. Effects of grafts of single anterior pituitary glands on the incidence and type of mammary neoplasm in neutron- or gamma-irradiated Fischer female rats. *Cancer Res.*, **36**, 3732–3735 (1976).

3. Furth, J. The role of prolactin in mammary carcinogenesis. *In* "Human Prolactin. International Congress Series No. 308," ed. J. L. Pasteels and C. Robyn, pp. 233–248 (1973). Excerpta Medica, Amsterdam.

4. Henderson, B. E., Gerkins, V., Rosario, I., Casagrande, J., and Pike, M. C. Elevated serum levels of estrogens and prolactin in daughters of patients with breast cancer. *New Engl. J. Med.*, **293**, 790–795 (1975).

5. Kanda, K., Kobayashi, T., Okamoto, K., and Shibata, T. Thermal neutron standard field with a marwellian distribution using the KUR heavy water facility. *Nucl. Instr. Methods*, **148**, 535–541 (1978).

6. Kim, U. and Furth, J. Relation of mammary tumors to mammotropes. II. Hormone responsiveness of 3-methylcholanthrene-induced mammary carcinomas. *Proc. Soc. Exp. Biol. Med.*, **103**, 643–645 (1960).

7. Montour, J. L., Hard, R. C., and Flora, R. E. Mammary neoplasia in the rat following high-energy neutron irradiation. *Cancer Res.*, **37**, 2619–2623 (1977).

8. Murray, R. M., Mozaffarian, G., and Pearson, O. H. Prolactin levels with L-Dopa treatment in metastatic breast carcinoma. *In* "Prolactin and Carcinogenesis," ed. A. R. Boyns and K. Griffiths, pp. 158–161 (1972). Cardiff, Wales: Alpha Omega Alpha.

9. Nagasawa, H. and Yanai, R. Effects of estrogen and/or pituitary grafts on nucleic acid synthesis of carcinogen-induced mammary tumors in rats. *J. Natl. Cancer Inst.*, **52**, 1219–1222 (1974).

10. Proceedings of US-Japan Joint Workshop for Reassessment of Atomic Bomb Radiation Dosimetry (1983). RERF, Hiroshima.

11. Proceedings of Second US-Japan Joint Workshop for Reassessment of Atomic Bomb Radiation Dosimetry (1984). RERF, Hiroshima.

12. Rolandi, E., Barreca, T., Masturzo, P., Polleri, A., Indiveri, F., and Barabino, A. Plasma-prolactin in breast cancer. *Lancet*, **2**, 845–846 (1974).

13. Segalof, A. and Maxifield, W. S. The synergism between radiation and estrogen in the production of mammary cancer in the rat. *Cancer Res.*, **31**, 166–168 (1971).

14. Shellabarger, C. J. Modifying factors in rat mammary gland carcinogenesis. *In* "Biology of Radiation Carcinogenesis," ed. J. M. Yuhas, R. W. Tennant, and J. D. Regan, pp. 31–43 (1976). Raven Press, New York.

15. Shellabarger, C. J., Brown, R. D., and Rao, A. R. Rat mammary carcinogenesis following neutron or x-radiation. *In* "Biological effects of neutron irradiation. IAEA symposium series," pp. 391–401 (1974). International Atomic Energy Agency, Vienna.

16. Shellabarger, C. J., Cronkite, E. P., Bond, V. P., and Lippincott, S. W. The occurrence of mammary tumors in the rat after sublethal whole-body irradiation. *Radiat. Res.*, **6**, 501–512 (1957).

17. Sheth, N. A., Ranadive, K. J., Suraiya, J. N., and Sheth, A. R. Circulating levels of prolactin in human breast cancer. *Br. J. Cancer*, **32**, 160–167 (1975).

18. Takizawa, S. Hormonal implication in initiation and progression of experimental mammary tumors in rats. *Acta Pathol. Jpn.*, **23**, 683–693 (1973).

19. Tokunaga, M., Land, C. E., Yamamoto, T., Asano, M., Tokuoka, S., Ezaki, H., Nishimori, I., and Fujikura, T. Breast cancer among atomic bomb survivors. *In* "Radiation Carcinogenesis: Epidemiology and Biological Significance," ed. J. D. Boice, Jr. and J. F. Fraumeni, Jr., pp. 45–56 (1984). Raven Press, New York.

20. Tokunaga, M., Norman, J. E., Asano, M., Tokuoka, S., Ezaki, H., Nishimori, I., and Tsuji, Y. Malignant breast tumors among atomic bomb survivors, Hiroshima and Nagasaki, 1950–74. *J. Natl. Cancer Inst.*, **62**, 1347–1359 (1979).

21. Tokuoka, S., Asano, M., Yamamoto, T., Tokunaga, M., Sakamoto, G., Hartmann, W. H., Hutter, R.V.P., Land, C. E., and Henson, D. E. Histologic review of breast cancer cases in survivors of atomic bombs in Hiroshima and Nagasaki, Japan. *Cancer*, **54**, 849–854 (1984).

22. Vogel, H. H., Jr. Mammary gland neoplasia after fission neutron irradiation. *Nature*, **222**, 1279–1281 (1969).

23. Vogel, H. H., Jr. and Zaldivar, R. Neutron-induced mammary neoplasms in the rat. *Cancer Res.*, **32**, 933–938 (1972).

24. Yokoro, K. and Furth, J. Relation of mammotropes to mammary tumors. V. Role of mammotropes in radiation carcinogenesis. *Proc. Soc. Exp. Biol. Med.*, **107**, 921–924 (1961).

25. Yokoro, K. and Furth, J. Determining role of "mammotropes" in induction of mammary tumors in mice by virus. *J. Natl. Cancer Inst.*, **29**, 887–909 (1962).

26. Yokoro, K., Furth, J., and Haran-Ghera, N. Induction of mammotropic pituitary tumors by X-rays in rats and mice. The role of mammotropes in development of mammary tumors. *Cancer Res.*, **21**, 178–186 (1961).

27. Yokoro, K., Nakano, M., Ito, A., Nagao, K., Kodama, Y., and Hamada, K. Role of prolactin in rat mammary carcinogenesis: Detection of carcinogenicity of low dose carcinogens and of persisting dormant cancer cells. *J. Natl. Cancer Inst.*, **58**, 1777–1783 (1977).

28. Yokoro, K., Sumi, C., Ito, A., Hamada, K., Kanda, K., and Kobayashi, T. Mammary carcinogenic effect of low-dose fission radiation in Wistar/Furth rats and its dependency on prolactin. *J. Natl. Cancer Inst.*, **64**, 1459–1466 (1980).

GANN Monograph on Cancer Research 32, 1986

LEUKEMIA, MULTIPLE MYELOMA, AND MALIGNANT LYMPHOMA

Michito Ichimaru,[*1] Takeshi Ohkita,[*2]
and Toranosuke Ishimaru[*3]

*Department of Internal Medicine, Atomic Disease Institute, Nagasaki
University School of Medicine,[*1] Department of Hematology,
Research Institute for Nuclear Medicine and
Biology, Hiroshima University,[*2] and
Department of Epidemiology and Statistics, Radiation
Effects Research Foundation[*3]*

Excess risk of leukemia among atomic bomb (A-bomb) survivors increased with radiation dose in Hiroshima and Nagasaki. The incidence of all types of leukemia, except chronic lymphocytic leukemia, has increased among A-bomb survivors. However, chronic myelogenous leukemia (CML) is thought to be the most characteristic type of the A-bomb induced leukemias.

The highest risk of leukemia among A-bomb survivors was recognized in 1951 and has not yet disappeared in survivors in Hiroshima. Excess risk of leukemia in the younger age at time of bomb (ATB) groups appeared early; however, in the older age ATB groups it appeared much later especially among Hiroshima survivors. In both cities the effect of radiation exposure on the occurrence of CML was more clearly observable in the younger age ATB groups and occurred more frequently in Hiroshima. Leukemia among individuals exposed in utero and children of A-bomb survivors has not increased significantly. The relationship between radiation induced leukemia and chromosome abnormalities is discussed.

Twenty years after the A-bomb, the risk of multiple myeloma (MM) increased among survivors aged 20–59 years ATB. Non-Hodgkin's malignant lymphoma also increased among A-bomb survivors and showed roughly the same tendency as MM.

The hematopoietic system is one of the most sensitive systems for exposure to radiation, and leukemia is considered an important disease as a late effect in atomic-bomb (A-bomb) survivors.

A significant increase of several kinds of cancer has been reported among survivors during the 38 years since the A-bomb in 1945 (*12, 22*). However, the occurrence of leukemia was clearly observable in the earliest period after the bomb. Leukemia data for A-bomb survivors have presented the most useful information about radiation induced leukemia. Among hematopoietic malignancies, multiple myeloma (MM), which

---

[*1] Sakamoto-machi 12-4, Nagasaki 852, Japan (市丸道人).

[*2] Kasumi 1-2-3, Minami-ku, Hiroshima 734, Japan; Present address: National Nagoya Hospital, 3-94-1-1 Nakaku, Nagoya 460, Japan (大北　威).

[*3] Hijiyama Park 5-2, Minami-ku, Hiroshima 732, Japan (石丸寅之助).

was not previously found to be significantly elevated in A-bomb survivors, has gradually increased in heavily exposed persons 20 years after the bomb. Anderson and Ishida (2) and Nishiyama *et al.* (18) have reported the incidence of malignant lymphoma in A-bomb survivors.

Recently many types of leukemia have been considered stem cell diseases. In A-bomb survivors the incidence of all types of leukemia, except chronic lymphocytic leukemia, has increased and consequently it is suggested that A-bomb radiation initially affected immature hematopoietic stem cells. However, MM is a malignant disease of differentiated B lymphocytes and malignant lymphoma is a disease of mature lymphocytes (usually T- or B-cells) as is chronic lymphocytic leukemia. Thus, the difference in prevalence and period of occurrence of these diseases in A-bomb survivors seems quite interesting in terms of the radiation effect on the hematopoietic system.

In this review, we would like to describe the occurrence and the characteristics of the hematological malignancies among A-bomb survivors and consider the relationship of these diseases to A-bomb radiation.

Estimation of radiation dose for each survivor is important for clarification of the radiation effect. So far, the tentative 1965 dose (T65D) estimates which were estimated in 1965 by Oak Ridge National Laboratory (17) have been used for dose estimation of each A-bomb survivor. However, dosimetry of A-bomb radiation in Hiroshima and Nagasaki is now being reassessed after the Lawrence Livermore National Laboratory reported revised A-bomb radiation estimates in 1981 (15). This means that the neutron dose in both cities, and especially in Hiroshima, will decrease in the new estimations. As no conclusion has yet been reached, the T65D was used in this review.

A Radiation Effects Research Foundation (RERF) fixed sample of 109,000 subjects (82,000 survivors and 27,000 controls) was used to show the relationship between the incidence of these diseases and A-bomb radiation effects.

Leukemia

Leukemia cases among A-bomb survivors estimated to have received a radiation dose greater than 1 rad increased gradually from 1946 with maximum occurrence ob-

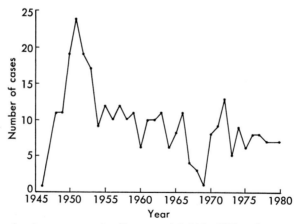

FIG. 1. Leukemia among proximally exposed (within 2000 m from ground zero) A-bomb survivors who received more than 1 rad radiation dose, Hiroshima and Nagasaki, 1945.

served in 1951, six years after the A-bomb. After 1951 the occurrence of leukemia decreased gradually with some fluctuation but there has been no year where the annual incidence among the proximally exposed (within 2,000 m from ground zero) was zero (Fig. 1). We would like to illustrate probable A-bomb induced leukemia using the RERF sample. A total of 189 leukemia cases (149 in Hiroshima and 40 in Nagasaki) have been detected during 1950–78 among these subjects.

Annual Incidence Rate for Leukemia by Dose, City, and Type of Leukemia

Figure 2 shows the crude annual incidence rate in the RERF sample during 1950–78 by dose, city, and two major types of leukemia, acute leukemia and chronic myelogenous leukemia (CML). Note, first, that the risk of all types of leukemia increases with dose in both cities, except for Nagasaki survivors who received less than 100 rad kerma total dose (average marrow total dose). Second, the risk of CML increases among individuals who received less than 50 rad kerma total dose in Hiroshima, but in Nagasaki the risk is significantly increased only among survivors who received 200 rad or more kerma total dose. The shape of the dose-response curves differs between the two cities and for acute leukemia and CML.

Annual Incidence Rate for All Types of Leukemia by Dose, City, Age at Time of Bomb (ATB), and Period

Figure 3 shows the trend of the standardized annual incidence rates for all types of leukemia by dose and city. The excess risk in individuals who received 200 rad or more

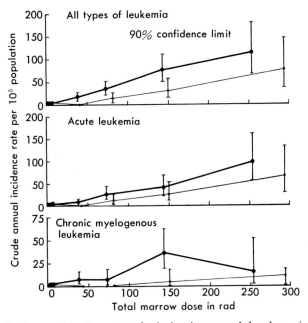

Fig. 2. Crude annual incidence rate for leukemia among A-bomb survivors in the RERF sample by total marrow dose, type of leukemia, and city, 1950–78. ●, Hiroshima; •, Nagasaki.

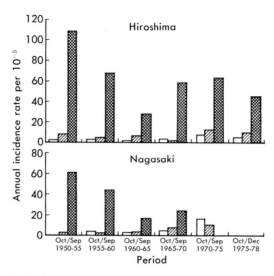

F<small>IG</small>. 3.   Standardized annual incidence rate for all types of leukemia in the RERF sample by dose, time period, and city, 1950–78. ☐, control; ▨, 1–99 rad; ▩, 100+ rad.

kerma total dose has declined with time after exposure in both cities. In Hiroshima the downward trend has been slow and the effect extends to 1978, but in Nagasaki the excess risk declined sharply with time after exposure and disappeared by 1970. Thus, the pattern of disappearance of the leukemogenic effect with time after exposure seems to differ by city. In Nagasaki, it seems very important to confirm whether or not the leukemogenic effect truly disappeared. The occurrence of leukemia in a so-called open sample of A-bomb survivors in Nagasaki was examined from 1970–78 and 2 or 3 leukemia cases per year were identified among those with exposure of 1 rad or more. Further, several cases of preleukemia were detected in the proximally exposed survivors since 1970 (4). In view of these facts, it may be inappropriate to say that the leukemogenic effect of A-bomb radiation has disappeared in Nagasaki, although it appears to have disappeared among the RERF sample in Nagasaki. One of the reasons for this apparent disappearance may be that the size of the RERF sample in Nagasaki is too small (15,000 survivors and 11,000 controls).

Kawakami *et al.* (*13*) reported 19 cases of leukemia that occurred during 1978–81 among A-bomb survivors who were exposed within 2,000 m from ground zero in Hiroshima and indicated that there still is a risk of A-bomb induced leukemia.

Figure 4 gives the age ATB specific annual incidence rate for all types of leukemia during 1950–78 by dose and city. The excess risk in individuals who received 100 rad or more kerma total dose did not differ significantly among four age ATB categories.

Figure 5 shows the age ATB specific annual incidence rate for all types of leukemia among individuals who received 100 rad or more kerma total dose by city and period. When the age ATB specific annual incidence rates are examined for dose and years after exposure, it is noted that the larger the excess risk among those of younger ages ATB who received 100 rad or more kerma total dose, the greater the effect of radiation in the early period and the more rapid the decline in risk up to 1960. The effect among those persons who were aged 30 years or more ATB is of lesser magnitude, but it is more

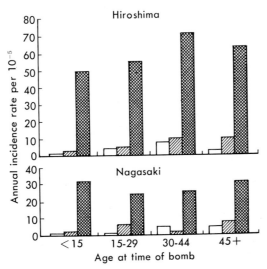

Fig. 4. Age ATB specific annual incidence rate for all types of leukemia in the RERF sample by dose, and city, 1950–78. □, control; ▨, 1–99 rad; ▩, 100+ rad.

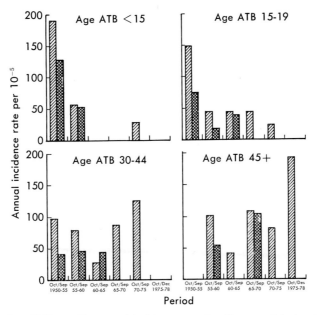

Fig. 5. Age ATB specific annual incidence rate for all types of leukemia among survivors who received 100 rad or more by time period and city, 1950–78. ▨, Hiroshima; ▩, Nagasaki.

prolonged. The effect among individuals who were aged 45 years or more ATB did not appear until 1955 (10 years after exposure) and the risk has been highest in the most recent 3 years in Hiroshima. The risk has been greater in Hiroshima than in Nagasaki for most age ATB groups and for most periods. After 1970, an excess risk in survivors in the RERF sample who received 100 rad or more kerma total dose is apparent in Hiroshima survivors whose age ATB was 30 or more. Again, the leukemogenic effect of

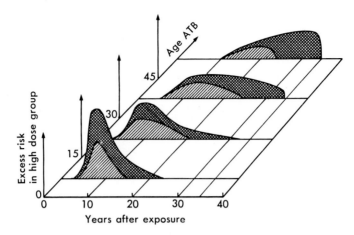

FIG. 6. Schematic diagram of the leukemogenic effect of A-bomb radiation by age ATB, elapsed years after exposure (latent period), and city. ■, Hiroshima; ▨, Nagasaki.

radiation in A-bomb survivors by age ATB, elapsed years after exposure, and city is given in Fig. 6.

Incidence of Leukemia by Subtype

Table I presents the age ATB specific incidence rates for leukemia among Hiroshima and Nagasaki survivors who received 100 rad or more kerma total dose by four age ATB groups, leukemia subtype, and four periods plus total period. As shown in the upper panel, the risk of acute myelogenous leukemia (AML) increases with age ATB, but the risk of acute lymphocytic leukemia (ALL) and CML was seen more frequently in the younger age group. The risk of AML and other acute leukemia (AL) except ALL has become greater in the older age ATB group only as time after exposure elapsed. After 1970, radiation seems effective for induction of only AML among those aged 45 years or more ATB. In the younger age group (less than 10 years old) there are few cases of AML, which occurs in all age groups. However, ALL among nonexposed individuals is more frequent in the younger age group. Accordingly, the occurrence of ALL seems to have decreased as time after exposure elapsed. CML in nonexposed persons is an adult leukemia and the fact that CML among A-bomb survivors was seen frequently in the younger age group and only in the early period suggests a strong radiation effect on the occurrence of CML which seems to be the most characteristic leukemia as a late effect of A-bomb radiation. Furthermore, CML occurred in Hiroshima survivors more frequently than in Nagasaki where only 10 cases of CML among A-bomb survivors were observed in the early period (CML total cases to 1975, 68 in Hiroshima and 15 in Nagasaki).

As stated above, there is some difference in the occurrence of leukemia among A-bomb survivors in the two cities. The difference is mainly the higher incidence of total leukemia and CML in Hiroshima. Ishimaru et al. (9) suggest that the difference was due to the larger dose of neutrons in Hiroshima according to the T65 dose estimates. However, the neutron dose is likely to decrease in the new estimation which raises the

TABLE I. Age ATB Specific Annual Incidence Rate (per 100,000) for Leukemia among
Survivors who Received 100 rad or More Kerma Total Dose, by Type of
Leukemia and Time Period, Hiroshima and Nagasaki, 1950–78

Type of Leukemia	Age ATB			
	< 15	15–29	30–44	45+
	Total period			
Person-years	41,326	54,559	32,205	19,011
CML	14.5 (6)	7.3 (4)	15.5 (5)	5.3 (1)
AML	2.4 (1)	12.8 (7)	27.9 (9)	36.8 (7)
ALL	12.1 (5)	9.2 (5)	6.2 (2)	5.3 (1)
AL	12.1 (5)	9.2 (5)	6.2 (2)	5.3 (1)
	October 1950–September 1955			
Person-years	7,545	10,060	6,489	5,346
CML	66.3 (5)	29.8 (3)	46.2 (3)	0.0 (0)
AML	0.0 (0)	39.8 (4)	30.8 (2)	0.0 (0)
ALL	53.0 (4)	29.8 (3)	0.0 (0)	0.0 (0)
AL	39.8 (3)	9.9 (1)	0.0 (0)	0.0 (0)
	October 1955–September 1960			
Person-years	7,429	9,908	6,230	4,516
CML	0.0 (0)	0.0 (0)	0.0 (0)	22.1 (1)
AML	13.5 (1)	0.0 (0)	64.2 (4)	44.3 (2)
ALL	13.5 (1)	10.1 (1)	0.0 (0)	0.0 (0)
AL	26.9 (2)	20.2 (2)	0.0 (0)	22.1 (1)
	October 1960–September 1970			
Person-years	14,597	19,349	11,485	6,446
CML	0.0 (0)	5.2 (1)	0.0 (0)	0.0 (0)
AML	0.0 (0)	10.3 (2)	26.1 (3)	46.5 (3)
ALL	0.0 (0)	5.2 (1)	8.7 (1)	15.5 (1)
AL	0.0 (0)	10.3 (2)	8.7 (1)	0.0 (0)
	October 1970–December 1978			
Person-years	11,755	15,242	8,001	2,703
CML	8.5 (1)	0.0 (0)	25.0 (2)	0.0 (0)
AML	0.0 (0)	6.6 (1)	0.0 (0)	74.0 (2)
ALL	0.0 (0)	0.0 (0)	12.5 (1)	0.0 (0)
AL	0.0 (0)	0.0 (0)	12.5 (1)	0.0 (0)

Number of cases in parentheses.
CML, Chronic myelogenous leukemia.
AML, Acute myelogenous leukemia.
ALL, Acute lymphocytic leukemia.
AL, Other type of acute leukemia.

problem of how to explain the difference in the occurrence of A-bomb induced leukemia
in the two cities.

Chronic Myelogenous Leukemia (CML)

Figure 7 shows the annual incidence rates for CML in each age ATB group. It is
apparent that CML in A-bomb survivors appeared early in the younger age group.
Thus, the leukemogenic effect of A-bomb radiation is more evident in CML than in
other types of leukemia and CML is thought to be the most characteristic A-bomb
radiation-induced human leukemia.

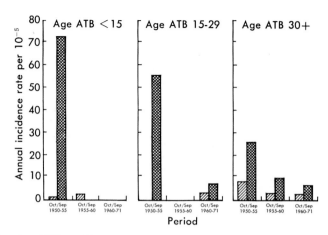

FIG. 7. Age ATB specific annual incidence rate (per 100,000 of CML among A-bomb survivors, by dose and time period, 1950–71. ▨, 1–99 rad; ▩, 100+ rad.

Typical CML with Ph¹ chromosome has not been observed in animal leukemia, so information about CML obtained from A-bomb survivors is important. Ph¹ chromosome was demonstrated in all CML patients among A-bomb survivors examined and there has been no clear difference between the features of CML among A-bomb survivors and nonexposed persons.

CML in A-bomb survivors could be found in the early phase without splenomegaly. After detailed observations of CML in A-bomb survivors, Kamada *et al.* (*11*) pointed out the progressive manifestations of CML as appearance of Ph¹ chromosome → increased basophils → elevated leukocytes → decrease of neutrophil alkaline phosphatase (NAP) → elevated serum VB_{12} → splenomegaly.

The Nishiyama district in Nagasaki is known as an area of A-bomb radioactive fallout and residents of Nishiyama were possibly exposed to low dose radiation externally as well as internally by means of the continuous intake of agricultural products during a long period. The estimated dose of only the external exposure in this area was reported to be 30 to 130 rad by Okajima. Leukocytosis of unknown cause was recognized about 2 years after the A-bomb (*5*). Later, two cases of CML occurred among residents of this area. Long-term exposure to low dose radiation is likely to induce CML.

Leukemia Among Individuals Exposed in Utero, and Children of A-Bomb Survivors

The incidence of leukemia has been analyzed in relation to the fetal dose of individuals exposed in utero, and the parental gonadal dose of individuals born to A-bomb survivors and controls in two RERF fixed samples (in utero mortality and clinical follow-up). Among 3,636 in utero exposed children and controls, 3 leukemia cases were identified through 1979 (*8*).

Table II shows the crude annual incidence rate for leukemia among the in utero exposed children and controls in Hiroshima and Nagasaki during 1945–79. There were 3 leukemia cases in this sample during the 34-year follow-up period. No excess risk for exposed children appears to exist. Only one person among those individuals who received 1 rad or more developed acute lymphocytic leukemia.

TABLE II. Crude Annual Incidence Rate for Leukemia among in Utero Exposed Children and Controls, Hiroshima and Nagasaki, 1945–79

Item	Fetus total dose in rad				Total
	NIC	0	1–49	50+	
Subjects	2,306	625	620	85	3,636
Person-years	72,444	19,403	19,078	2,255	113,180
Leukemia cases	1	1	1	0	3
Rate (10^{-5})	1.38	5.15	5.24	0.00	2.65
90% confidence limit Upper	6.55	24.46	24.87	—	6.85
Lower	0.07	0.27	0.27	—	0.72

Leukemia Cases

No.	MF No.	Sex	Fetus dose		Type of leukemia	Onset	Age at onset	Date of birth
			Gamma	Neutrons				
1	848523	M	2 rad	0	Acute lymphocytic	March 1976	29	1 April 1946
2	246505	F	0	0	Acute myelogenous	July 1963	18	8 August 1945
3	442671	M	NIC		Acute, type undetermined	December 1954	9	7 December 1945

TABLE III. Crude Annual Incidence Rate for Leukemia in the F_1 Mortality Sample by Parental Gonadal Dose, Hiroshima and Nagasaki, 1946–79

Maternal dose in rad	Item	Paternal dose in rad			Total
		50+	1–49	Control[a]	
50+	Subjects	177	129	2,035	2,341
	Person-years	4,673	3,394	52,942	61,009
	Case	0	1	1	2
	Rate (10^{-5})	0.0	29.5	1.9	3.3
	90% confidence limits Upper	—	139.8	9.0	10.3
	Lower	—	1.5	0.1	0.6
1–49	Subjects	401	1,703	7,291	9,395
	Person-years	10,678	46,983	193,926	251,587
	Case	0	0	4	4
	Rate (10^{-5})	0.0	0.0	2.1	1.6
	90% confidence limits Upper	—	—	4.7	3.6
	Lower	—	—	0.7	0.5
Control*	Subjects	1,713	3,264	33,976	38,953
	Person-years	44,361	85,379	897,043	1,026,783
	Case	2	2	26	30
	Rate (10^{-5})	4.5	2.3	2.9	2.9
	90% confidence limits Upper	14.2	7.4	4.0	4.0
	Lower	0.8	0.4	2.0	2.1
Total	Subjects	2,291	5,096	43,302	50,689
	Person-years	59,712	135,756	1,143,911	1,339,379
	Case	2	3	31	36
	Rate (10^{-5})	3.3	2.2	2.7	2.7
	90% confidence limits Upper	10.6	5.7	3.7	3.6
	Lower	0.6	0.6	2.0	2.0

[a] 0 rad + not in city ATB.

Table III gives the crude annual incidence rate for leukemia among children born to exposed parents and controls in the F_1 mortality samples, Hiroshima and Nagasaki, by parental gonadal dose. In this sample 36 leukemia cases have been identified during 1946–79. There is no significant excess risk among these children where either or both parents were exposed.

Based on retrospective studies of children exposed in utero or the preconception exposure of their parents to diagnostic X-rays, a significant increased risk of leukemia in the in utero exposed and children conceived subsequent to exposure has been reported by Stewart et al. (19), McMahon (14), and Graham et al. (3). However, studies of A-bomb survivors show no significant excess risk of leukemia among in utero exposed children nor among children born to exposed parents.

Radiation Induced Leukemia and Chromosome Abnormality

The study of chromosomes seems to be one useful method to clarify the mechanism of radiation effects on leukemogenesis as leukemia is a disease of monoclonal proliferation of white blood cells. Even now some healthy A-bomb survivors have chromosome abnormalities in peripheral blood lymphocytes in proportion to their estimated radiation dose. Kamada (10) and Tomonaga (21) reported a significant increase of chromosome abnormalities in bone marrow cells of A-bomb survivors, and specific chromosome abnormalities have been identified in several types of leukemia. It may be possible to clarify the mechanism of radiation induced leukemia by studying the relationship of chromosome abnormalities among healthy A-bomb survivors and survivors with leu-

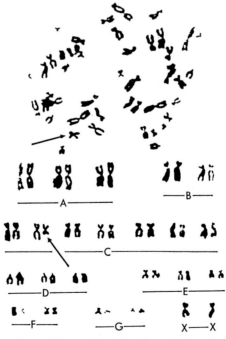

FIG. 8. Karyotype detected from colony-forming unit in culture (CFU-C) colony of proximally exposed A-bomb survivor having chromosome abnormality with 46xy, cq- (probable 7q-)

kemia. Tanaka *et al.* (*20*) reported that the chromosome break points of the T-lympho-cytes of healthy A-bomb survivors are nonrandom, and relatively frequent abnormalities were observed in specific break points. The same chromosome abnormality (7q-) was found in one proximally exposed healthy survivor and a preleukemia case (probable chronic myelomonocytic leukemia) in another proximally exposed survivor (Fig. 8). Recently, Amenomori *et al.* (*1*) established a method of chromosome analysis using colony forming cells induced from hematopoietic stem cells. This method is considered useful to identify whether or not the same chromosome abnormalities seen in peripheral lymphocytes of A-bomb survivors also exist in their hematopoietic stem cells. In addition, it will be possible by this method to elucidate whether or not specific chromosome abnormalities in leukemia patients are also present in their hematopoietic stem cells.

Multiple Myeloma (MM)

MM is a malignancy of B-cell (plasma cell) lineage and is a relatively rare disease. Malignant cells in this disease proliferate mainly in the bone marrow. The incidence of MM among A-bomb survivors previously had not been found to be significantly elevated. On the basis of Atomic Bomb Casualty Commission (ABCC) autopsy material for 1948–62 Anderson and Ishida (*2*) reported that the incidence of MM among A-bomb survivors in Hiroshima was slightly increased in the group exposed within 1,400 m from ground zero, as compared to the incidence in those individuals exposed beyond that distance; however, there was only one MM case in the group exposed within 1,400 m. Yamamoto and Wakabayashi (*23*) reported an absence of evidence of radiation induced bone tumors, including MM, in A-bomb survivors in Hiroshima and Nagasaki during 1950–65. Nishi-yama *et al.* (*18*) also studied malignant lymphoma and MM in the same fixed sample of A-bomb survivors, but they could not demonstrate a significant excess risk of MM

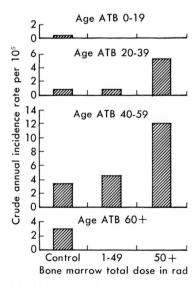

FIG. 9. Crude annual incidence rate of multiple myeloma for A-bomb survivors and controls in the RERF sample, by age ATB and total marrow dose, Hiroshima and Nagasaki, 1950–76.

in the heavily exposed. Thus, for 20 years after the A-bombs, no persuasive evidence of an excess of MM among the survivors was found.

In 1982, more than 30 years after the A-bombs, an analysis of MM incidence was conducted among A-bomb survivors and controls for the 26-year period from October 1950 to December 1976 and 29 cases of MM were identified (6). These 29 cases were divided into 3 bone marrow total dose classes (50+ rad, 1–49 rad, and controls) and 4 age ATB groups (0–19, 20–39, 40–59, and 60+). As shown in Fig. 9, the relative risk in those aged 20 to 59 years ATB tends to increase with dose for both sexes in both cities. When the data were divided into the 3 dose groups and 4 age ATB groups, the number of cases in each of the 12 categories was small. However, a dose effect was not evident among those individuals whose age ATB was less than 20 years or 60 or more years, although the risk tends to increase in the control group with age.

Clearly, MM occurs frequently after 50 years of age, and thus the failure to see an effect in the under 20 years group may merely reflect the fact that these individuals have not yet reached the age at which MM is more prone to develop. The apparent absence of a radiation effect among the older individuals is thought to be due to other reasons.

The size of the oldest group was small especially in the heavily exposed, and most of these individuals may have died before MM would have occurred as a radiation effect. A dose effect for MM was evident only among those individuals 20–59 years of age ATB. Observation of the under 20 age ATB group when they have reached the age of risk is suggested.

A simple graphical method called "hazard plotting" was used to compare the cumulative risk of MM in 3 dose groups in relation to years after exposure. Figure 10 shows the cumulative hazard rates for individuals aged 20–59 ATB in 3 marrow dose groups from 1950 to 1976. An increased risk in the high-dose group (50+ rad) does not

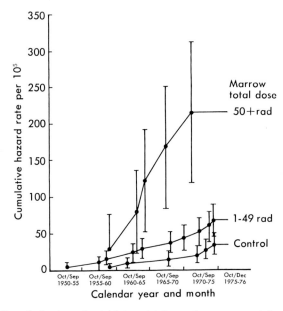

FIG. 10.   Cumulative hazard rate for multiple myeloma among A-bomb survivors and controls aged 20–59 years ATB in the RERF sample, Hiroshima and Nagasaki, 1950–76.

become apparent until 20 years after exposure when the risk shows a gradual increase.

As myelomatous cells are of B-lymphocyte lineage, MM, like malignant lymphoma, seems to be a malignancy of mature lymphocytes. The carcinogenic effect for blood cells seems to differ in their differentiated level. Furthermore, some age-dependent factor may be necessary for the occurrence of MM.

The risk of MM for the under age 20 ATB group may develop in the future, and a significant increase in malignant monoclonal M-protein disease (MM and macroglobulinemia) 35 years after exposure has been confirmed again using the RERF Life Span Study (LSS) sample during October 1979–September 1981 (16).

Malignant Lymphoma

Anderson and Ishida (2) reported excess risk of malignant lymphoma including Hodgkin's disease, lymphosarcoma, reticulum cell sarcoma, and MM among Hiroshima A-bomb survivors using autopsy and surgical materials during 1949–62. Nishiyama *et al.* (18) also reported the same findings among Hiroshima survivors using the materials during 1945–65. The incidence of malignant lymphoma except MM was reviewed using the RERF sample during 1950–77. Table IV gives the prevalence rate of malignant lym-

TABLE IV. Prevalence Rate for Malignant Lymphoma in the RERF Sample by Dose and Type of Lymphoma, Hiroshima and Nagasaki, 1950–77

| Item | Dose category (rad) | | | | | |
	Control (A)	1–99 (B)	100–199 (C)	200+ (D)	Unknown	Total
Number of subjects	41,028	39,204	3,111	2,930	2,409	88,682
Average total dose (rad)	0	17.3	141.2	349.6	—	
			Number of cases			
Hodgkin's disease	10	10	2	0	0	22
Non-Hodgkin's lymphoma	45	41	3	9	1	99
Malignant lymphoma (total)	55	51	5	9	1	121
		Crude prevalence rate per 1,000 population				
Hodgkin's disease	0.24	0.26	0.64	0.00	0.00	0.25
Non-Hodgkin's lymphoma	1.10	1.05	0.96	3.07	0.42	1.12
Malignant lymphoma	1.34	1.31	1.60	3.07	0.42	1.37
Standardized relative risk	1.0	1.0	1.3	2.6		

A=(C+D) $\chi^2(1)=3.361$ $p<0.10$ suggestive.
A=(D) $\chi^2(1)=5.594$ $p<0.05$ significant.

TABLE V. Relationship between Age ATB and Year of Onset for Malignant Lymphoma Cases in the LSS Sample Who Received 200 rad or More Radiation Dose

| Year of onset | Age ATB | | | | |
	0–19	20–39	40–59	60+	Total
−1950	1	0	0	0	1
1951–1960	0	1	0	1	2
1961–1970	1	2	1	0	4
1971–1977	0	2	0	0	2
Total	2	5	1	1	9

phoma in the sample by dose and type of lymphoma for Hiroshima and Nagasaki.

The crude prevalence rate of non-Hodgkin's lymphoma among survivors exposed to 200 rad or more showed a significant increase. However, there was no increase of Hodgkin's disease among A-bomb survivors. There were more malignant lymphoma cases who received 200 rad or more detected since 1960 as shown in Table V. It appears that non-Hodgkin's lymphoma increased after 1960 as well as MM.

Recently, malignant lymphoma has been divided into T- or B-cell types by surface marker study of tumor cells. It would be interesting to learn which type of malignant lymphoma was induced by A-bomb radiation. In Kyushu, the predominant occurrence of T-cell type non-Hodgkin's lymphoma was reported (7). Surface marker data are not available for study of these cases among A-bomb survivors.

REFERENCES

1. Amenomori, T., Tomonaga, M., Tomonaga, Y., Yao, E., Jinnai, I., Yoshida, Y., Kuriyama, K., Matsuo, T., Sadamori, N., and Ichimaru, M. A simple method for chromosomal preparation from individual hematopoietic colonies. *Acta Haematol. Jpn.*, **46**, 665–670 (1983) (in Japanese).

2. Anderson, R. E. and Ishida, K. Malignant lymphoma in the survivors of the atomic bomb in Hiroshima. *Ann. Intern. Med.*, **61**, 853–862 (1964).

3. Graham, S., Levin, M. L., Lilienfeld, A. M., Schuman, L. M., Gibson, R., Dowd, J. E., and Hempleman, L. Preconception, intrauterine, and postnatal irradiation as related to leukemia. *Natl. Cancer Inst. Monogr.*, **19**, 347–371 (1966).

4. Ichimaru, M. The diseases of hematopoietic organs among A-bomb survivors, Nagasaki. *Clinika*, **8**, 981–989 (1981) (in Japanese).

5. Ichimaru, M. Late effects of atomic bomb radiation in the Nishiyama district. *Hiroshima Igaku*, **29**, 294–297 (1976) (in Japanese).

6. Ichimaru, M., Ishimaru, T., Mikami, M., and Matsunaga, M. Multiple myeloma among atomic bomb survivors in Hiroshima and Nagasaki, 1950–76: Relationship to radiation dose absorbed by marrow. *J. Natl. Cancer Inst.*, **69**, 323–328 (1982).

7. Ichimaru, M., Kinoshita, K., Kamihira, S., Ikeda, S., Yamada, Y., and Amagasaki, T. T-cell malignant lymphoma in Nagasaki district and its problems. *Jpn. J. Clin. Oncol.*, **9** (Suppl.), 337–346 (1979).

8. Ishimaru, T., Ichimaru, M., and Mikami, M. Leukemia incidence among individuals exposed in utero, children of atomic bomb survivors and their controls: Hiroshima and Nagasaki, 1945–1979. RERF Tech. Rep. 11-81 (1981).

9. Ishimaru, T., Otake, M., and Ichimaru, M. Dose relationship of neutron and gamma rays to leukemia incidence among atomic bomb survivors in Hiroshima and Nagasaki by type of leukemia, 1950–1971, *Radiat. Res.*, **77**, 377–394 (1979).

10. Kamada, N. The atomic bomb and cancer—from the standpoint of chromosome aberrations. *Nagasaki Med. J.*, **47**, 356–366 (1972) (in Japanese).

11. Kamada, N., Oguma, N., Tanaka, R., Kuramoto, A., Ohkita, T., Takahashi, H., Ito, C., and Kimura, H. Development of chronic myelocytic leukemia in atomic bomb survivors. *Hiroshima Igaku*, **33**, 506–511 (1978) (in Japanese).

12. Kato, H. and Schull, W. J. Studies of the mortality of A-bomb survivors. 7, Mortality, 1950–78, Part 1. Cancer mortality. *Radiat. Res.*, **90**, 395–432 (1982).

13. Kawakami, M., Hayakawa, N., Tanaka, K., Ohkita, T., and Kurihara, N. Recent trends of A-bomb leukemia in Hiroshima, 1972–1981, and two cases of early CGL diagnosed among proximally exposed survivors. *Hiroshima Igaku*, **3**, 477–480 (1984) (in Japanese).

14. MacMahon, B. Prenatal X-ray exposure and childhood cancer. *J. Natl. Cancer Inst.*, **28**, 1178–1191 (1962).
15. Marshall, E. New A-bomb studies alter radiation estimates. *Science*, **212**, 900–903 (1981).
16. Mikami, M., Ishimaru, T., Kuramoto, A., Abe. T., Yamada, Y., Amagasaki, T., and Ichimaru, M. M-proteinemia in A-bomb survivors and controls, Hiroshima and Nagasaki, Oct. 1979– Sept. 1981. RERF Tech. Rep., in preparation.
17. Milton, R. C. and Shohoji, T. Tentative 1965 radiation dose estimation for atomic bomb survivors, Hiroshima and Nagasaki. ABCC Tech. Rep. 1-68 (1968).
18. Nishiyama, H., Anderson, R. E., Ishimaru, T., Ishida, K., Ii, Y., and Okabe, N. The incidence of malignant lymphoma and multiple myeloma in Hiroshima and Nagasaki atomic bomb survivors, 1945–65. *Cancer*, **32**, 1301–1309 (1973).
19. Stewart, A., Webb, J., and Hewitt, D. A survey of childhood malignancies. *Br. Med. J.*, **1**, 1495–1508 (1958).
20. Tanaka, K., Kamada, N., Ohkita, T., and Kuramoto, A. Chromosome break points in T-lymphocytes from atomic bomb survivors: Comparison with specific chromosome aberrations found in leukemia. *Hiroshima Iagaku*, **35**, 1214–1221 (1982) (in Japanese).
21. Tomonaga, Y. Chromosome abnormalities in atomic bomb survivors. *Nagasaki Med. J.*, **51**, 282–286 (1976) (in Japanese).
22. Watanabe, S. Cancer and leukemia developing among atom-bomb survivors, Geshwulste, Tumors I (Handbuch der allgemeinen Pathologie, Vol. 5), ed. by E. Grundmann, pp. 461–577 (1974). Springer-Verlag, Berlin.
23. Yamamoto, T., and Wakabayashi, T. Bone tumors among the atomic bomb survivors of Hiroshima and Nagasaki. *Acta Pathol. Jpn.*, **19**, 201–212 (1969).

CANCER OF THE THYROID AND SALIVARY GLANDS

Haruo EZAKI,[*1] Toranosuke ISHIMARU,[*2] Yuzo HAYASHI,[*3]
and Nobuo TAKEICHI[*4]

*Department of Clinical Studies, Radiation Effects Research Foundation,[*1]
Department of Epidemiology and Statistics, Radiation Effects Research
Foundation,[*2] Asa Citizens' Hospital[*3], and Second Department
of Surgery, Hiroshima University School of Medicine[*4]*

The relationship of atomic bomb (A-bomb) exposure to tumors of the head and neck has been studied in detail for the thyroid and salivary gland.

Thyroid. It has been demonstrated by animal experiments and studies conducted on those undergoing radiation therapy of the neck during childhood, and on those exposed to radioactive fallout from Hydrogen-bomb tests in the Marshall Islands, that thyroid neoplasms can be induced by radiation. Under the assumption that A-bomb radiation would have a similar effect, interest has focussed on the A-bomb survivors from an early stage. From the 1950s, reports were made on such cases suspected to have been induced by the A-bomb. From the 1960s, systematic analyses have been conducted primarily on the development of thyroid cancer in the Atomic Bomb Casualty Commission-Radiation Effects Research Foundation (ABCC-RERF) Adult Health Study (AHS) sample. The number of detected thyroid cancer cases has increased with time. The conclusion of these studies indicated that the incidence of thyroid cancer is high among A-bomb survivors, being remarkably so in those exposed within 1,500 m from ground zero. Similar findings have been observed in patients of the Hiroshima University School of Medicine and of the national health insurance program. Since the sample size for the earlier studies was small with only a few thyroid tumor cases, Ezaki studied the incidence of clinical thyroid cancer and occult thyroid cancer in Hiroshima during 1958–79 using the ABCC-RERF Life Span Study (LSS) sample composed of 75,493 subjects. The results of this study showed the incidence of clinical cancer to be higher, the greater the dose, this tendency being especially predominant in females exposed at young ages. The incidence of occult cancer primarily detected by autopsy was significantly higher in those exposed to 50+ rad than in the control group.

Salivary gland. Although it was assumed that radiation would have a similar effect on the salivary gland located near the thyroid gland, it was only in the 1970s that studies were commenced on the salivary gland.

Takeichi *et al.* in their statistical study of salivary gland tumor cases diagnosed at hospitals in Hiroshima and Kure, and Belsky *et al.* in their study of the AHS population observed a high incidence of salivary

[*1] Hijiyama Park 5-2, Minami-ku, Hiroshima 732, Japan (江崎治夫).
[*2] Hijiyama Park 5-2, Minami-ku, Hiroshima 732, Japan (石丸寅之助).
[*3] Nakashima Kabe-cho 1810, Asakita-ku, Hiroshima 731–02, Japan (林　雄三).
[*4] Kasumi 1-2-3, Minami-ku, Hiroshima 734, Japan (武市宣雄).

gland cancer among A-bomb survivors. In a subsequent study on the AHS population the incidence of salivary gland tumors was 9.3-fold higher in the group exposed to 300+ rad than in the control group and when confined only to malignant tumors the incidence was 21.8-fold higher.

Thyroid

Reports on thyroid cancer in Hiroshima and Nagasaki atomic bomb (A-bomb) survivors can be traced back to the 1950s. Kaneko and Numata (*10*) reported in 1957 a case of thyroid cancer which developed with leukemia in a 12-year old girl exposed to A-bomb radiation at a distance of 800 m from ground zero in Hiroshima, and in 1959 Fujimoto *et al.* (*5, 6*) reported three cases of thyroid cancer in A-bomb survivors.

In 1963 Hollingsworth *et al.* (*8*) made a systematic analysis of thyroid gland diseases in a population of survivors and suggested the presence of a tendency for the incidence of thyroid cancer to be high among A-bomb survivors. They studied 12 thyroid cancer cases found in the AHS population during 1958–59 and suggested that the incidence of thyroid cancer was high among proximally exposed (within 1,500 m from ground zero) survivors, especially among females. The study was continued on the same population, and Socolow *et al.* (*14*), making an analysis in 1963 on 21 cases of thyroid cancer identified during the 3-year period 1958–61, confirmed that the incidence of thyroid cancer was high among A-bomb survivors proximally exposed. Wood *et al.* (*19*) reported similar results in 1968, in which they studied the relationship between radiation dose and thyroid cancer incidence among survivors exposed within 2,000 m from ground zero and demonstrated a tendency for the incidence to be elevated with increased dose. Parker *et al.* (*11*) summarized a 1958–71 study on the same population. According to their summarization, the number of cases of thyroid cancer identified during this period was 74, and the incidence was high in the 50+ rad group, especially in females exposed at under 20 years of age. Of the 74 cases 34 were found only at postmortem examination. Minute cancer was found at a high frequency at autopsy, and it is known that most such cancer does not develop into malignancies which would become clinically apparent. If the analysis is made including minute cancer found at autopsy, the incidence will become elevated but no longer be applicable to clinical experience.

Members of the LSS sample, a larger ABCC-RERF study population, are included in the ABCC-RERF autopsy program. During 1957–68 autopsies were conducted on 3,067 cases, and Sampson *et al.* (*12, 13*) made detailed examinations on the thyroid glands of these cases and found thyroid cancer in 536 cases. Of these cases 518 (96.6%) were occult cancer less than 1.5 cm in size. Analysis of these 536 cases showed increased thyroid cancer prevalence in A-bomb survivors exposed to 50+ rad.

Reports have been made on thyroid cancer among survivors studied in other study populations, but these are not fixed populations. Ezaki and Shigematsu (*3*) studied the incidence of thyroid cancer in patients seen in the outpatient clinic of the Department of Surgery, Hiroshima University School of Medicine, and found it to be 2.25% (38/1,509) and significantly higher in those exposed to A-bomb radiation as compared to 0.44% (58/13,211) for the nonexposed. The incidence of thyroid cancer in the exposed was higher in females, with 32 of 38 cases being females as against 6 males. Six of the 38 cases (15.8%) were A-bomb survivors proximally exposed within 1,000 m from ground zero indicating that thyroid cancer incidence is high among them. Further, 7 of the 38 cases were so-called early entrants who entered the city within two weeks after the bombing.

Ezaki and Shigematsu (3) studied thyroid cancer incidence among those insured under the national health insurance program in Hiroshima City during 1960–61 in order to observe the tendency in Hiroshima City as a whole, and the incidence in A-bomb survivors (26.80 per 100,000 population) was found to be almost 5-fold that in the nonexposed (5.25 per 100,000 population). Harano et al. (7) studied 394 cases of thyroid gland diseases operated on and histopathologically diagnosed in Nagasaki City by 1965 and found 116 cases of thyroid cancer. Since 42 of these cases were exposed to the A-bomb and 74 were controls (43.6% exposed and 24.8% nonexposed) they reported that thyroid cancer incidence was higher in the exposed.

Among the study samples established to date, ABCC-RERF studies have been made mainly on the sample composed of 20,000 AHS subjects, but this population is small for conducting epidemiological studies. On the other hand, the populations of other studies have the disadvantage of not being fixed populations and having no radiation dose estimation made for them. Overcoming these disadvantages, Ezaki (4) studied and analyzed data on thyroid cancer diagnosed or detected at autopsy during the 22 years from 1958 to 1979, in a sample of 75,493 study subjects exposed in Hiroshima belonging to the LSS Extended sample, excluding those whose exposure dose was unknown and those who had thyroid cancer from before 1958.

In past studies, clinically detected thyroid cancer and occult (minute) thyroid cancer were reported together, but in this study they are discussed separately because they differ greatly in character. There were 332 subjects in the population suspected of having thyroid cancer, and they were examined individually for identification. As a result, 125 cases of clinical thyroid cancer and 159 cases of occult thyroid cancer were detected.

1. Clinical thyroid cancer

The histopathological distribution of the 103 cases for which tissue specimens were obtained is shown in Table I. Most were papillary cancer, with no difference by exposure status. The 125 cases were composed of 15 males and 110 females, distributed by age at the time of the bomb (ATB) and exposure dose, as shown in Table II and Fig. 1;

TABLE I. Distribution of Histological Type of Clinical Thyroid Cancer Cases Whose Tissue Specimens were Obtained, Hiroshima, 1958–79

Morphologic type of carcinoma	Tissue total dose in rad			
	Control	1–49	50+	Total
Papillary	43 (100.0)	38 (90.5)	16 (88.9)	97 (94.2)
Sclerosing	0	0	0	0
Follicular	0	2 (4.8)	1 (5.6)	3 (2.9)
Epidermoid	0	1 (2.4)	0	1 (1.0)
Anaplastic	0	1 (2.4)	1 (5.6)	2 (2.0)
Medullary	0	0	0	0
Total	43 (100.0)	42 (100.1)	18 (100.1)	103 (100.1)

Percentage in parentheses.

TABLE II.   Crude Annual Incidence Rates for Clinical Thyroid Cancer per 100,000
Population by Sex and Tissue Total Dose, Hiroshima 1958–79

Item	Thyroid tissue total dose in rad				
	Control	1–49	50–99	100+	Total
			Male		
Subjects	18,842	9,977	797	798	30,414
Average dose	0.0	9.1	71.2	205.6	—
Person-years	351,551	184,857	14,259	14,245	564,912
Cases	9	3	2	1	15
Rate (10^{-5})	2.6	1.6	14.0	7.0	2.7
			Female		
Subjects	28,200	14,578	1,182	1,119	45,079
Average dose	0.0	10.1	69.2	197.2	—
Person-years	554,902	284,995	23,143	21,840	884,880
Cases	46	48	7	9	110
Rate (10^{-5})	8.2	16.8	30.2	41.2	12.4

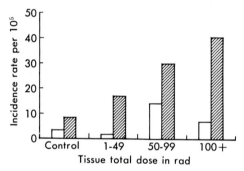

FIG. 1.   Crude annual incidence rates for clinical cancer per 100,000 population by
sex and tissue total dose. □, male ; ▨, female.

and the crude annual incidence per 100,000 population was 2.7 for males and 12.4 for
females. The risk of thyroid cancer in females and in both sexes combined increased
with increase of dose. The increase in the high dose group is not remarkable in males,
but this may be due to their small number. In males too the trend is for risk to increase
with radiation dose, but this trend is not statistically significant, given the small number
of cases. In females the crude annual incidence rate shows an increase of risk with increase of dose in every age group, and this tendency was particularly evident in those
exposed at a young age (Table III).

When observed and expected numbers were calculated and ratios of observed to
expected (O/E) sought, either by sex or sexes combined, the incidence of thyroid cancer
was found to increase with increased dose. When tests of linear response were made by
Mantel's statistical method to determine the presence or absence of a dose effect, a
statistically significant relation was observed in females and in males and females combined. No relation could be demonstrated in males because there were few male thyroid
cancer cases (Table IV). The O/E ratio showed a tendency to increase with exposure
dose in every age ATB group, and this was especially remarkable in those under 20 years
of age. Tests of linear response, which shows dose effect, showed it to be statistically

TABLE III. Age ATB Specific Annual Incidence Rates for Clinical Thyroid Cancer by Tissue Total Dose and Sex, Hiroshima 1958–79

Age ATB	Item	Male — Tissue total dose in rad					Female — Tissue total dose in rad				
		Control	1–49	50–99	100+	Total	Control	1–49	50–99	100+	Total
0–9	PY[a]	100,210	51,009	3,067	2,647	156,933	103,048	52,737	3,445	2,994	162,224
	Cases	1	0	0	1	2	4	5	1	1	11
	Rate (10^{-5})	1.00	0.00	0.00	37.78	1.27	3.88	9.48	29.03	33.40	6.78
10–19	PY	90,006	48,884	3,494	4,185	146,569	118,766	57,500	5,626	5,903	187,795
	Cases	3	0	1	0	4	8	9	2	4	23
	Rate (10^{-5})	3.33	0.00	28.62	0.00	2.73	6.74	15.65	35.55	67.76	12.25
20–29	PY	31,554	16,403	1,322	1,851	50,930	105,998	55,155	4,984	4,920	171,057
	Cases	3	0	0	0	3	16	6	1	1	24
	Rate (10^{-5})	9.51	0.00	0.00	0.00	5.89	15.10	10.88	20.06	20.33	14.03
30–39	PY	48,864	24,389	2,399	2,011	77,663	104,156	55,255	3,903	3,771	167,085
	Cases	1	1	0	0	2	6	12	1	2	21
	Rate (10^{-5})	2.05	4.10	0.00	0.00	2.58	5.76	21.72	25.62	53.04	12.57
40–49	PY	53,129	28,279	2,664	2,257	86,329	80,170	42,132	3,572	3,193	129,065
	Cases	1	1	0	0	2	9	11	1	1	22
	Rate (10^{-5})	1.88	3.54	0.00	0.00	2.32	11.23	26.11	28.00	31.34	17.05
50+	PY	27,989	15,893	1,313	1,293	46,488	42,763	22,215	1,612	1,063	67,854
	Cases	0	1	1	0	2	3	5	1	0	9
	Rate (10^{-5})	0.00	6.29	76.16	0.00	4.30	7.02	22.51	62.04	0.00	13.30
Total	PY	351,552	184,857	14,259	14,244	554,912	554,901	234,995	23,142	21,842	884,880
	Cases	9	3	2	1	15	45	48	7	9	110
	Rate (10^{-5})	2.55	1.62	14.03	7.02	2.66	8.29	16.84	30.25	41.21	12.43

Both sexes

		Control	1–49	50–99	100+	Total
Total	PY	906,453	469,852	37,401	35,086	1,449,792
	Cases	55	51	9	10	125
	Rate (10^{-5})	6.07	10.85	24.06	27.71	8.62
	Standardized incidence rate (10^{-5})	5.62	10.02	25.42	20.30	7.92

Standard incidence rate adjusted for sex and age ATB.

[a] Person-years.

TABLE IV.   Comparison of Observed and Expected Number of Clinical Thyroid
Cancer Cases by Tissue Total Dose and Sex, Hiroshima 1958–79

Item	Tissue total dose in rad					Test for linearity χ^2 [1] p
	Control	1–49	50–99	100+	Total	
Average dose in rad	0	9.7	70.0	200.7	—	
			Total			
Subjects	47,042	24,555	1,979	1,917	75,493	
Observed	55	51	9	10	125	26.46
Expected	78.05	40.53	3.28	3.14	125.00	$p<0.001$***
O/E	0.70	1.26	2.74	3.18	1.00	
			Male			
Subjects	18,843	9,977	797	798	30,414	
Observed	9	3	2	1	15	2.70
Expected	9.30	4.90	0.40	0.40	15.00	$p<0.10$ NS
O/E	0.97	0.61	5.00	2.50	1.00	
			Female			
Subjects	28,200	14,578	1,182	1,119	45,079	
Observed	46	48	7	8	110	23.81
Expected	68.75	35.63	2.88	2.74	110.00	$p<0.001$***
O/E	0.67	1.35	2.43	3.28	1.00	

Expected number adjusted for age ATB.
NS (Not significant), $0.10<p$; $0.05<p\leqslant0.10$; * $0.01<p\leqslant0.05$; ** $0.001<p\leqslant0.01$; *** $p\leqslant0.001$.

TABLE V.   Comparison of Observed and Expected Number of Clinical Thyroid Cancer
Cases by Tissue Total Dose and Age ATB, Hiroshima 1958–79

Item	Tissue total dose in rad					Test for linearity χ^2 [1] p
	Control	1–49	50–99	100+	Total	
Average dose in rad	0	9.7	70.0	200.7	—	
		Age ATB: under 20				
Subjects	19,060	9,733	731	745	30,274	
Observed	16	14	4	6	40	34.64
Expected	25.27	12.69	1.02	1.02	40.00	$p<0.001$***
O/E	0.63	1.10	3.92	5.88	1.00	
		Age ATB: 20–39				
Subjects	14,084	7,355	609	627	22,575	
Observed	26	19	2	3	50	2.88
Expected	31.03	16.30	1.32	1.35	50.00	$0.10<p<0.05$
O/E	0.84	1.17	1.52	2.22	1.00	
		Age ATB: 40 and over				
Subjects	13,398	7,462	639	545	22,544	
Observed	13	18	3	1	35	1.91
Expected	21.75	11.54	0.94	0.77	35.00	$p>0.10$ NS
O/E	0.60	1.56	3.19	1.30	1.00	

Expected number adjusted for sex

significant in those under age 20 ATB, suggestive in those 20–39, and unclear in those
40 and over, with dose effect more evident the younger the age (Table V). The relative
risk of thyroid cancer in the 50+ rad group as compared to the control group and the

TABLE XII.   Incidence of Salivary Gland Tumors by Age ATB and
Exposure Distance, Hiroshima 1953–71

| Exposure distance | Age in years | | | | | |
| | 0–19 | | 20–49 | | 50+ | |
	Cases	Incidence	Cases	Incidence	Cases	Incidence
0–1,500 m	5	4.9	8	4.2	1	2.2
1,501–5,000 m	4	1.0	8	1.4	5	3.4
5,000+m (nonexposed)	19	0.6	10	0.7	1	1.3

Crude incidence per 100,000 per year.

annual incidence per 100,000 population for the exposed cases in Hiroshima was 1.9 which is 2.7-fold higher than the 0.7 for the 30 nonexposed cases, and for the early entrants it was 1.4 which is 2-fold higher than that of the nonexposed. The difference was more apparent for malignant tumors, the incidence for the directly exposed cases being 10-fold higher and that for the early entrants being 6-fold higher than that for the nonexposed cases (Table X). Classified by exposure distance into cases proximally exposed within 1,500 m from ground zero, cases distally exposed at 1,500–5,000 m, and cases nonexposed at more than 5000 m, the annual incidence per 100,000 population was 3.8 for the proximally exposed, 1.3 for the distally exposed, and 0.7 for the nonexposed, with the incidence showing a tendency to be higher the closer to ground zero. The tendency was marked in the malignant tumors (Table XI). Studying the relationship to exposure distance by age ATB, the incidence of salivary gland tumors in those 19 and under and 20–49 was found to show a tendency to increase with decrease of exposure distance, the crude incidence being a very high 4.9 per year per 100,000 population in those proximally exposed at age 19 and under ATB (Table XII). The histopathological diagnoses of all salivary gland tumors collected by Takeichi et al. (15, 17, 18) are shown by exposure in Table XIII.

Since 8 cases detected in the study belonged to the population reported previously by Belsky et al. (1), Belsky et al. (2) made a reanalysis of the 30 salivary gland tumor cases in the fixed population adding these 8 cases. As a result, it was found that the incidence rate for salivary gland tumors was high among those exposed to 300+ rad, and that the relative risk was compared to their controls (those not in the city (NIC) ATB and the 0 rad exposed) was as high as 9.35, and that for malignant tumors taken alone was a high 21.8 (Table XIV).

TABLE XIII. Histological Type of Salivary Gland Tumors 1950–71

Tumor	Exposed cases					Nonexposed cases				
	Parotid	Sub-maxillary	Sub-lingual	Minor	Total	Parotid	Sub-maxillary	Sub-lingual	Minor	Total
Benign tumor	26 [1]	5	0	0	31 [1]	66 (12) [10]	21 (6) [3]	0	6 (3) [1]	93 (21) [14] [(1)]
Benign mixed tumor	18	4	—	—	22	57 (10) [10]	21 (6) [3] [(1)]	—	6 (3) [1]	84 (19) [14] [(1)]
Papillary cystadanomata lymphomatosa	5	1	—	—	6	6 (1)	—	—	—	6 (1)
Oxyphilic adenoma	—	—	—	—	—	2	—	—	—	2
Other adenoma	1 [1]	—	—	—	1 [1]	— (1)	—	—	—	(1)
Benign lymphoepithelial lesion	2[a] [1]	—	—	—	2	1	—	—	—	1
Malignant tumor	17	9	1	4	31	19 (1) [3]	7 [1]	2 [1]	3	31 (1) [5]
Malignant mixed tumor	5	4	1	1	11	5	2	1 [1]	1	9 [1]
Mucoepidermoid tumor	5	1	—	1	7	6 (1) [1]	2 [1]	1	—	9 (1) [2]
Squamous cell carcinoma	1	1	—	—	2	2 [1]	—	—	—	2 [1]
Adenocarcinoma	1	3	—	1	5	2	1	—	1	4
Adenoid cystic	1	—	—	1	2	1	1	—	—	2
Acinic cell	—	—	—	—	—	1	1	—	—	2
Mucous cell	4	—	—	—	4	2 [1]	—	—	1	3 [1]
Miscellaneous form	—	—	—	—	—	—	—	—	—	—
Total	43 [1]	14	1	4	62 [1]	85 (13) [13]	28 (6) [4] [(1)]	2 [1]	9 (3) [1]	124 (22) [19] [(1)]

( ) Tumor cases in persons born after the A-bomb.

[ ] Tumor cases in residents outside of Hiroshima Prefecture.

[a] Bilateral case developed in one patient.

TABLE XIV. Salivary Gland Neoplasms Following Atomic Radiation

Item	Tentative 1965 dose in rad			Total
	NIC+0	1–299	300+	
Population	57,859	40,457	1,340	99,656
Person-years	700,552	487,669.5	16,171.5	1,204,393
All cases				
Observed	14	13	3	30
Expected	17.45	12.15	0.40	30.00
Relative risk	1.00	1.33	9.35	
Malignant cases				
Observed	4	3	2	9
Expected	5.23	3.64	0.12	9.00
Relative risk	1.00	1.08	21.8	

REFERENCES

1. Belsky, J. L., Tachikawa, K., Cihak, R. W., and Yamamoto, T. Salivary gland tumors in atomic bomb survivors, Hiroshima-Nagasaki, 1957–1970. *J. Am. Med. Assoc.*, **219**, 864–868 (1972).

2. Belsky, J. L., Takeichi, N., Yamamoto, T., Cihak, R. W., Hirose, F., Ezaki, H., Inoue, S., and Blot, W. J. Salivary gland neoplasms following atomic radiation: Additional cases and reanalysis of combined data in a fixed population, 1957–1970. *Cancer*, **35**, 555–559 (1975).

3. Ezaki, H. and Shigemitsu, T. Studies on thyroid cancer induced by A-bomb exposure and its clinical characteristics. *J. Hiroshima Med. Assoc.*, **20** (Suppl.), 336–347 (1967); *Proc. Hiroshima Univ. Res. Inst. Nucl. Med. Biol.*, **11**, 166–168 (1970) (in Japanese).

4. Ezaki, H. Thyroid carcinoma after exposure to atomic bomb radiation, Hiroshima 1958–79. *J. Jpn. Pract. Surg. Soc.*, **44**, 1127–1137 (1983) (in Japanese).

5. Fujimoto, Y., Yamamoto, T., Numata, J., and Mori, K. Two autopsy cases of thyroid cancer in young atomic bomb survivors. *J. Hiroshima Med. Assoc.*, **12**, 519–524 (1959) (in Japanese).

6. Fujimoto, Y., Yamamoto, T., Ishida, J., and Numata, J. Three autopsy cases of myelogenous leukemia complicated with thyroid gland tumors detected in atomic bomb survivors. *J. Hiroshima Med Assoc.*, **12**, 1077 (1959) (in Japanese).

7. Harano, A., Tezuka, H., and Shirabe, R. Thyroid gland—Study of thyroid gland diseases in atomic bomb survivors. *J. Hiroshima Med. Assoc.*, **20** (Suppl.), 336–347 (1967) (in Japanese).

8. Hollingsworth, D. R., Hamilton, H. B., Tamagaki, H., and Beebe, G. W. Thyroid disease: A study in Hiroshima, Japan. *Medicine*, **42**, 47–71 (1963).

9. Ishimaru, T., Ezaki, H., Asano, M., Fujikura, T., Nishida, T., and Izumi, M. Incidence of thyroid cancer among atomic bomb survivors and controls, Hiroshima and Nagasaki, 1958–1979: Relationship to radiation dose absorbed by thyroid gland. (unpublished data).

10. Kaneko, N. and Numata, J. An autopsy case of atomic radiation-induced leukemia complicated with thyroid gland tumor. *J. Pediatr. Pract.*, **20**, 478 (1957) (in Japanese).

11. Parker, L. N., Belsky, J. L., Yamamoto, T., Kawamoto, C., and Keehn, R. J. Thyroid carcinoma after exposure to atomic radiation: A continuing survey of a fixed population, Hiroshima and Nagasaki, 1958–1971. *Ann. Intern. Med.*, **80**, 600–604 (1974).

12. Sampson, R. J., Key, C. R., Buncher, C. R., and Iijima, S. Thyroid carcinoma in Hiro-

shima and Nagasaki, I. Prevalence of thyroid carcinoma at autopsy. *J. Am. Med. Assoc.*, **209**, 65–70 (1969).

13. Sampson, R. J., Key, C. R., Buncher, C. R., Oka, H., and Iijima, S. Papillary carcinoma of the thyroid gland, sizes of 525 tumors found at autopsy in Hiroshima and Nagasaki. *Cancer*, **25**, 1391–1393 (1970).

14. Socolow, E. L., Hashizume, A., Neriishi, S., and Niitani, R. Thyroid carcinoma in man after exposure to ionizing radiation. A summary of the findings in Hiroshima and Nagasaki. *New Engl. J. Med.*, **268**, 406–410 (1963).

15. Takeichi, N., Inoue, S., Niimoto, M., Nagata, N., and Ezaki, H. Parotid gland tumors, especially in relation to radiation exposure. *J. Jpn. Surg. Soc.*, **74**, 1170–1172 (1973) (in Japanese).

16. Takeichi, N., Hirose, F., Inoue, S., Niimoto, M., and Hattori, T. Parotid gland tumors observed at Research Institute for Nuclear Medicine and Biology, Hiroshima Univeristy. *Jpn. J. Cancer Clin.*, **22**, 307–311 (1976) (in Japanese).

17. Takeichi, N., Hirose, F., and Yamamoto, H. Salivary gland tumors in atomic bomb survivors, Hiroshima, Japan. I. Epidemiologic observations. *Cancer*, **38**, 2462–2468 (1976).

18. Takeichi, N., Hirose, F., Yamamoto, H., Ezaki, H., and Fujikura, T. Salivary gland tumors in atomic bomb survivors, Hiroshima, Japan. II. Pathologic study and supplementary epidemiologic observations. *Cancer*, **52**, 377–385 (1983).

19. Wood, J. W., Tamagaki, H., Neriishi, S., Sato, T., Sheldon, W. F., Archer, P. G., Hamilton, H. B., and Johnson, K. G. Thyroid carcinoma in atomic bomb survivors, Hiroshima and Nagasaki. *Am. J. Epidemiol.*, **89**, 4–14 (1969).

MALIGNANT TUMORS IN ATOMIC BOMB SURVIVORS WITH SPECIAL REFERENCE TO THE PATHOLOGY OF STOMACH AND LUNG CANCER

Tsutomu Yamamoto,[*1] Issei Nishimori,[*2] Eiichi Tahara,[*3] and Ichiro Sekine[*2]

*Department of Pathology, Radiation Effects Research Foundation,[*1]*
Department of Pathology, Atomic Disease Institute, Nagasaki
*University School of Medicine,[*2] and Department of Pathology,*
*Hiroshima University School of Medicine[*3]*

A general review of stomach and lung cancer among atomic bomb (A-bomb) survivors is made classified by three time periods, 1945–60, 1960–75, and 1975–84. First is the period of "what is A-bomb disease?," during the second period the fixed population samples and the tentative 1965 radiation dose (T65D) estimates were established, and during the third period the tumor and tissue registries were operating and reassessment of radiation dose was underway. From review of stomach and lung cancer studies during the three time periods the following findings can be summarized: 1) the incidence of stomach and lung cancer among A-bomb survivors is related to radiation exposure dose, and the incidence of cancer increases at the usual ages when cancer appears, 2) cancer incidence is high among survivors who were exposed when young and the latent period is short, and 3) there is no specific histological type of radiation-induced cancer, but poorly differentiated types develop with a high frequency.

Of diseases suffered by atomic bomb (A-bomb) survivors in Hiroshima and Naga-saki, correlation with radiation dose has so far been observed only for malignant tumors, while for other diseases no such finding has been noted (*22*). Thus, it is important to focus interest on carcinogenesis due to A-bomb radiation not only for the welfare of survivors but also in ascertaining the mechanism of radio-carcinogenesis. This also means that the results of radiation-induced cancer in animal experiments may be an indication of similar effects in man. A-bomb survivors in Hiroshima and Nagasaki are the only large-scale population ever to experience whole-body exposure to a single dose of ionizing radiation.

In studying whether malignant tumors which developed in survivors are due to radiation or not, because radiation-induced cancers are not generally different from those otherwise present, it is necessary that epidemiological and statistical methods be used in comparative studies between findings of the exposed and nonexposed. Therefore, the following two requirements are essential: 1) definition of an exposed population, and 2) establishment of the radiation dose. Unfortunately, these two criteria have not yet been made even 39 years after the bombing. This has made it difficult to provide a clarifying

---

[*1] Hijiyama Park 5-2, Minami-ku, Hiroshima 732, Japan (山本　務).

[*2] Sakamoto-machi 12-4, Nagasaki 852, Japan (西森一正, 関根一郎).

[*3] Kasumi 1-2-3, Minami-ku, Hiroshima 734, Japan (田原栄一).

explanation for the so-called "A-bomb disease" which was used during the early years of studies on late A-bomb effects.

The study of cancer in survivors can be classified into the following three periods, the first period (1945–60), the second period (1960–75), and the third period (1975–84). During the first period, attention was focussed on the high incidence of leukemia and related disorders, but the study sample had not been well defined and all reports on exposure conditions were based on distance from ground zero, the tentative 1957 dose (T57D) estimates (4). During the second period, a fixed population consisting of approximately 100,000 subjects called the Life Span Study (LSS) sample was established in Hiroshima and Nagasaki by the Atomic Bomb Casualty Commission (ABCC) and the Japanese National Institute of Health (JNIH) (18). The T57D was revised and replaced with the tentative 1965 dose (T65D) (26) which was based on nuclear explosion tests in the US, and included individual exposure doses calculated with consideration given to shielding factors, whereas T57D was estimated from the air dose. The Unified Program was initiated based on three major programs, the Adult Health Study (AHS), the Pathology Study, and the LSS (7).

During the third period, the ABCC / Radiation Effects Research Foundation (RERF) Autopsy Study was phased out and Tumor Registries were established in Hiroshima and Nagasaki. Reassessment of radiation dose is also being made with new dose estimate expected in 1986. During the third period, attention began to be focussed on the occurrence of solid tumors other than leukemia.

Studies on the so-called "A-bomb disease" from the time of the A-bomb are extensive and diversified in scale and summarization will be attempted with the exception of certain periods which have been reported by others (9, 12, 15, 41). We would like primarily to describe stomach cancer and lung cancer, a statistical summarization will be made first, after which reports will be made on each cancer.

The First Period

During the first period, studies were conducted by Obo (33), Beebe et al. (5), Ishida (17), Harada et al. (14), and Shimizu (36, 37). In an attempt to resolve the question of "What is A-bomb disease?" Obo (33) classified 34,871 death certificates in Hiroshima from August 1945 to December 1959 by address, sex, age, and disease, and calculated the mortality rate for A-bomb survivors and the entire population of Hiroshima City. The mortality rate for survivors approximates the national average but is higher than the average for Hiroshima City and Prefecture. The shorter the distance from ground zero, the higher was the mortality. Obo stated that this was due to increased deaths from malignant neoplasms and that there were no other diseases of high frequency. Also in males, the mortality rates for stomach and lung cancer were higher than the national average.

Beebe et al. (5) reviewed the mortality rate for 1950–59 in the approximately 20,000 subjects of the AHS sample, a subsample of the LSS sample, and found that there was a relationship between radiation and leukemia, but not other causes of death.

In order to ascertain the state of development of malignant tumors in A-bomb survivors, the Hiroshima City Medical Association initiated a Tumor Registry program in Hiroshima City in May 1957 and in 1958 the Nagasaki City Medical Association started a registry in Nagasaki City. Ishida (17) and Harada et al. (14) compiled data for the 20 month period following initiation of the registry, in which it is shown that the morbidity rate of malignant neoplasms in survivors in 1957 and 1958 was higher closer to ground zero and the observed value within 1,000 m from ground zero was four times higher than the expected value. The ratio of the observed value to the expected value within 1,500 m from ground zero was 1.93 for stomach cancer and 4.31 for lung cancer.

Shimizu (36, 37) in distinguishing A-bomb survivors from the nonexposed on the basis of holders of the A-bomb Survivor's Health Handbook in Hiroshima City attempted a comparison between the two groups from 1957–60 with the use of vital statistics death schedules, and observed that the number of deaths due to malignant tumors was large within 2,000 m from ground zero, but no difference was seen between recognized A-bomb patients and non-A-bomb handbook holders. Shigeto (35) in studying, by distance from ground zero and age, 83 stomach cancer cases and 44 lung cancer cases seen among 39,404 outpatients (36,514 in the Department of Internal Medicine and 2,890 in the Department of Surgery) at the Hiroshima A-bomb Hospital from September 1956 to August 1963, obtained similar findings.

In a review of 175 malignant tumor cases among 580 cases autopsied during 1953–65 at the Hiroshima Prefectural Hospital, Monzen and Kikuchi (28) studied the relation of radiation to malignant neoplasms. They observed that malignant tumors were more frequent in relatively aged survivors within 2,000 m from ground zero, but due to the small number of survivors the relationship of specific malignant tumors and histological characteristics to radiation could not be ascertained. In a review of malignant tumors among survivors during 20 years post-bomb, Nishimori et al. (32) conducted an analysis of 4,619 cases autopsied at the Nagasaki University School of Medicine and observed radiation effects by distance from ground zero, but could not demonstrate any specific findings related to radiation. Angevine and Jablon (2) and Angevine et al. (3) reviewed diseases peculiar to survivors among 2,450 cases autopsied at Hiroshima and Nagasaki during 1948–59, but could not detect malignant tumors related to radiation except for leukemia and thyroid cancer. They observed that studies on late A-bomb effects based on autopsy cases require statistical consideration and that in the accumulation of cases epidemiological bias in the autopsy cases should be excluded as much as possible. No statistical significance was demonstrated in the relation of radiation to stomach and lung cancer. Zeldis et al. (48) obtained results suggestive of radiation carcinogenesis, but they could not demonstrate any relation between cancer of specific organs and radiation dose.

The Second Period

Ciocco (11) studied cumulative mortality rates from October 1950 to August 1964 for members of the LSS sample who were over 50 years of age as of October 1950, by exposure distance (more than 1,400 m and less than 1,400 m from ground zero). In this study lung cancer mortality rate was higher in those within 1,400 m with a significant difference in males. Stomach cancer mortality tended to be higher in those exposed 1,400 m but no significant difference was observed. However, he noted that the relative risk was high for 1950–55. With the use of death certificates for 1958–64 in Nagasaki, Mitani and Kidera (27) studied 3,481 malignant tumor cases assigned International Classification of Diseases (ICD 7th edition) code 140–205 to determine the difference in malignant tumors, if any, between exposed and nonexposed persons. The mortality due to malignant tumors in exposed persons was two to three times higher than in the nonexposed and higher than the national corrected mortality rate. These findings, he noted, indicate that radiation effects should not be ignored, but he could not demonstrate any specific tumor which was elevated in incidence only in the exposed. The incidence of malignant tumors was observed to be high among young persons exposed at 20–30 years of age in both sexes.

Many reports have been made on the ABCC fixed population from the middle of the second period (1960–75) to the third period (1975–84). Beebe *et al.* (*6*) reported that of 2,539 ABCC autopsy cases for 1950–65 in Hiroshima and Nagasaki, 225 cases were exposed within 1,400 m from ground zero and that, applying the estimated radiation dose, a significant relationship between radiation dose and malignant tumors among the autopsy cases was observed for lung cancer and leukemia but the finding was only suggestive for bladder cancer and urinary tract cancer. In a mortality study (*8*), he described that the relationship was suggestive for respiratory cancer and not significant for digestive cancer. Maki *et al.* (*23*) using data of 66 lung cancer cases detected among the AHS sample during 1950–66 reported an elevated risk of lung cancer, thyroid cancer, and breast cancer.

In a mortality study for the period 1950–70, Jablon and Kato (*21*) reported mortality in the high dose radiation group to be larger than in the low dose group and the not-in-city at the time of the bomb (ATB) group. They indicated that specific malignant tumors related to radiation were leukemia and all malignant tumors, but the relation was weak for uterine cancer and stomach cancer. The lung cancer rate was significantly higher in the group exposed to 100 rad or more than those exposed to 0–9 rad, especially in males. Only 10 of the 1,600 deaths from stomach cancer were among those aged 0–9 ATB and, although the two cases that occurred in the 200 rad group were more than 15 times the expected rate, generally the relationship to radiation could not be defined. By period, a significant difference was observed for 1965–70 but not for other periods. Even when these mortality studies were extended to 1972 (*29*), the relationship between stomach cancer, which accounted for approximately 40% of deaths in the sample, and ionizing radiation could not be clarified. The autopsy rate in the LSS sample reached 40% at the early stage, but it decreased gradually to 25% by 1970. It was reported (*38*) that the relationship to radiation was not significant in any cancer except for certain types of cancer and the relationship cannot be demonstrated by autopsy diagnosis alone.

The Third Period

ABCC-RERF has periodically reported on mortality from malignant tumors among survivors on the basis of death certificates. According to the recent report of Kato and Schull (*22*) for the period up to 1982, the mortality due to leukemia has continued to decrease with a difference from that in the controls observed only in Hiroshima. Contrary to this, an increase was observed in mortality from solid tumors among the survivors. They observed that malignant tumors developed at a higher rate at the time corresponding to the spontaneous development period and that both relative risk and absolute risk tended to be higher the younger the age ATB. According to mortality studies, the malignant tumor sites at present found to be significantly related to radiation dose are lung, breast, stomach, esophagus, urinary tract, colon, and myeloma, and it was after 1980 that a relationship was observed between stomach cancer mortality and radiation.

Stomach Cancer

It has gradually become evident that epidemiological and statistical consideration is necessary in the study of carcinogenesis among A-bomb survivors, but during the early and middle stages of studies on the late radiation effects, attempts were made to determine the morphological specificity of stomach cancer among A-bomb survivors. Since stomach cancer is the most frequent malignant tumor among the Japanese, it is quite natural that attempts were made to elucidate such specificity.

Imai *et al.* (*16*) employed 24 surgical cases and 9 autopsy cases of stomach cancer among A-bomb survivors in Hiroshima and Nagasaki and, as controls, stomach cancer cases (62 autopsy cases and 132 surgical cases) examined at the Department of Pathology, Kyushu University, with the aim of ascertaining the frequency of stomach cancer among A-bomb survivors and changes in host (A-bomb survivors) response to cancer. In their study of stomach cancer they could not demonstrate any difference between the survivors and the controls for histological type, developmental patterns, and postoperative course. Murphy and Yasuda (*30*) studied age at onset, age at initial examination, survival period, site of development, histological type, *etc.*, using 533 surgical and autopsy cases of stomach cancer (187 exposed cases) observed at ABCC in Hiroshima from December 1948 to June 1957. In their study, those exposed within 2,500 m from ground zero were regarded as A-bomb survivors, but no difference in stomach cancer was observed between the exposed group and the nonexposed group. Since the late effects of radiation on tissue are nonspecific, it is considered difficult to determine the morphological difference between the exposed and the nonexposed. Autopsy cases are selective and in particular during the early stage the selection was not statistically random and thus autopsy cases of stomach cancer were not considered to be representative of all deaths due to stomach cancer. It was thus difficult to determine the difference only through the findings obtained from autopsy cases and clinical cases. In order to elucidate the difference, it is necessary to compare all cases of stomach cancer diagnosed in Hiroshima City and Nagasaki City including exposed cases.

Uraki (*39*) studied by sex, age, site of development, histological findings, metastasis, *etc.*, 639 cases of stomach cancer (111 exposed and 402 nonexposed) diagnosed from January 1955 to December 1964, at Hiroshima University but could not demonstrate any difference between the exposed and nonexposed cases. Yamamoto *et al.* (*43–45*) attempted a pathohistological study on a total of 535 cases consisting of mainly autopsy and some surgical cases of stomach cancer belonging to the fixed populations in Hiroshima and Nagasaki during 1961–68, 1961–69, and 1961–74. Though some of the histological types (*i.e.*, tubular medullary, scirrhous, and mucocellular) tended to be most frequent in the heavily exposed survivors, no relationship between stomach cancer as a whole and exposure dose could be observed. Nakamura (*31*) studied stomach cancer cases appearing on death certificates of those belonging to the fixed populations in Hiroshima and Nagasaki for the period 1950–73 with emphasis on the heavily exposed and observed that although the number of stomach cancer cases decreased with increase in exposure dose, the mortality rate in Hiroshima increased with dose to peak at 400–499 rad. The relationship with dose was weaker in Nagasaki than in Hiroshima, but the highest mortality rate was observed at 500 rad. Although the collection of death certificates with stomach cancer as cause of death is nearly 100% complete, the reliability of such diagnosis is limited. In case of stomach cancer in the LSS population during 1961–75, the confirmation rate

TABLE I.   Incidence Rate and Relative Risk for Stomach Cancer by
Radiation Dose, Hiroshima and Nagasaki, 1950–77

Item	T65D in rad					
	Total	0	1–49	50–99	100–199	200+
Stomach cancer	2,155	832	1,010	113	92	108
Annual incidence ($\times 10^5$)	113.7	111.2	111.9	112.5	123.2	155.6
Relative risk	—	1.0	1.0	1.0	1.1	1.6***
Person-years ($\times 10^3$)	1,895.6	748.3	902.7	100.5	74.7	69.4

*** $p < 0.001$.

TABLE II.   Relative Risk for Stomach Cancer by Age ATB and Radiation Dose

Age ATB	T65D in rad				
	0	1–49	50–99	100–199	200+
0–9	1.0	0.7	0.6	1.1	4.2*
10–19	1.0	1.3	2.2	2.6	3.8***
20–29	1.0	1.1	1.5	1.4	2.2***
30–39	1.0	0.9	0.8	1.0	1.4
40–49	1.0	1.0	0.9	1.1	1.4*
50+	1.0	1.1	1.0	1.0	1.1

* $p < 0.05$,   *** $p < 0.001$.

(rate of clinical diagnosis confirmed by autopsy diagnosis) was 84.2% while the detection rate (rate of autopsy findings diagnosed clinically) was 75.6% (46). Attempts have been made to clinically detect stomach cancer patients by the cellular antibody technique, but since experimental techniques have not been established sufficiently, the relationship with dose has not yet been observed (1).

Matsuura et al. (25) recently collected as many stomach cancer cases in Hiroshima and Nagasaki as possible (2,155 cases diagnosed during 1950–77) and observed a statistically significant difference in the relationship with exposure dose. Confining themselves to the RERF LSS sample, they studied cases of clinical diagnosis, surgical cases, autopsy cases, and death certificate cases, and made full use of the tumor and tissue registries of the two cities. With regard to cases which had not been registered, they visited hospitals and clinics in the community in order to check the medical charts and collected 2,155 cases (1,720 in Hiroshima and 435 in Nagasaki) during 1955–77 and a histological review was made on 1,148 cases (53.3%). Table I shows the relative risk for stomach cancer cases by estimated exposure dose, using 1.0 as the relative risk for the 0 rad group. A significant ($p < 0.001$) relationship with stomach cancer cases was observed in the 200+ rad group (Table I). When stomach cancer cases are divided by age ATB, the relative risk is significantly high in those less than 30 ATB group (Table II). The time period from radiation exposure to development of stomach cancer is shortest in the 50 and over age ATB group, but there is no difference by radiation dose in each age group. Although there is no specificity in the site of development of stomach cancer in A-bomb survivors, classification of histological types shows that well differentiated adenocarcinoma and poorly differentiated adenocarcinoma tend to be frequent in stomach cancer in those with low radiation dose and those with high radiation dose, respectively (Table III).

TABLE III. Histological Type of Stomach Cancer, by Radiation Dose

Histological type		T56D in rad				
		Total	0	1–99	100–199	200+
Well differentiated adenocarcinoma	Observed	451	189	241	7	14
	%	45.2	48.8	46.8	17.1	25.6
Poorly differentiated adenocarcinoma	Observed	346	122	183	19	22
	%	34.7	31.5	35.5	46.3	40.7
Mucinous adenocarcinoma	Observed	57	28	21	3	5
	%	5.7	7.2	4.1	7.3	9.3

It is noteworthy that this study has demonstrated a relationship between stomach cancer in A-bomb survivors and exposure dose, a high incidence of stomach cancer in those less than 30 ATB, and that poorly differentiated adenocarcinoma tended to be the most frequent type. Clinically, Ito et al. (20) detected 43 stomach cancer cases in a mass X-ray stomach examination of survivors conducted during 1971–82, and, making a comparison between 3,369 cases whose doses had been determined and 3,819 cases who were more than 3,000 m from ground zero, observed a relationship between stomach cancer and radiation dose in those exposed to 100+ rad.

Lung Cancer

Lung cancer has a high incidence ranking next in order to stomach cancer. Different from gastric cancer, it had been assumed from early days that lung cancer was associated with exposure to radiation. Comprehensive research began from the second period (1960–75) during which a comparatively large number of cases were accumulated.

Fujimoto (13) studied the relationship of sex, age, and histological type by distance from ground zero among 50 lung cancer cases (32 male and 18 female) who were treated as outpatients of the Hiroshima A-bomb Hospital from September 1956 through August 1965. He surmised that there was a correlationship between lung cancer and A-bomb radiation in that there were 26 cases within 2,000 m from ground zero, 9 cases beyond 2,000 m and 15 cases among the proximally exposed (within 1,500 m from ground zero). Yamada (42) reviewed 31 lung cancer cases autopsied at Hiroshima University during 1960–65 on the basis of sex, age, radiation exposure, histological type, etc. The age at death of all cases was over 50, and 23 cases (74.1%) were between age 60–79. There were 13 A-bomb survivors exposed at 1,000–2,000 m from ground zero of whom 9 had squamous cell carcinoma. Importance is being attached to internal irradiation through inhalation of residual radioactive substances as a cause of lung cancer among A-bomb survivors.

During 1950–60, a study of lung cancer in the LSS sample was conducted by Wanebo et al. (40). Lung cancer cases were collected through clinical diagnosis, the tumor registry, autopsy records, and death certificates, and it was strongly suggested that lung cancer incidence increased with radiation dose. Although lung cancer frequency among A-bomb survivors exposed to 90 rad was higher than the expected value, no difference in age at onset, histological type, and other epidemiological factors was observed with the control group. Mansur et al. (24) reviewed the same sample pathologically and conducted an analysis of 200 lung cancer cases autopsied during 1950–64, when the autopsy rate was high (about 40%). Although a significant increase in lung cancer incidence was observed among A-bomb survivors exposed to 128 rad or more, no histological type specific to lung cancer of A-bomb survivors has yet been found. Cihak *et al.* (*10*) carried out studies during 1961–70 after more autopsy cases had been accumulated. The relationship with radiation was determined for 204 (5.4%) lung cancer cases among 3,778 autopsy cases in the LSS sample and the histological type was classified according to the WHO Histological Classification. Lung cancer cases among A-bomb survivors exposed to 200 or more rad were compared with those exposed to less than 1 rad, and the former had an incidence twofold greater. Classification by histological type showed 39 cases (19.1%) were of small cell anaplastic type and there was a significant increase among the 200 or more rad group. The fact that lung cancer of small cell anaplastic type was found at high frequency among A-bomb survivors is a finding similar to a report at the time that many uranium mine workers also had the same type of lung cancer, and thus it was interpreted that this type was a specific type of radiation lung cancer.

It is important to exclude environmental factors other than radiation considered to cause malignant tumors in A-bomb survivors, but it is difficult to do so. Review of the relationship between lung cancer in A-bomb survivors and smoking should be made. Although Ishimaru *et al.* (*19*) attempted to elucidate the effects of radiation and smoking on lung cancer incidence by interviewing 198 pairs composed of confirmed lung cancer cases and their controls, a definite conclusion could not be made. Concerning this problem, Kato and Schull (*22*) state that radiation and smoking have an additive relation with lung cancer incidence, that is, each of them is independently associated with the incidence, but another report (*34*) indicates that it is impossible to identify whether the relationship is additive or multiplicative (the factors interacting with each other).

Yamamoto (*47*) collected 1,057 lung cancer cases from the LSS sample in Hiroshima and Nagasaki during 1950–80 through clinical diagnosis, surgical cases, autopsy diagnosis, death certificates, *etc.* He studied the relationship between lung cancer and exposure dose using the revised T65D, and also tried to classify histologically the 488 cases available for review. The incidence of lung cancer in the 100 or more rad exposed group in both Hiroshima and Nagasaki was significantly higher than that for their control 0 rad group and the same results were obtained from cases confirmed histologically (Table IV). This finding was observed in both males and females. Review by age ATB showed each age group with an exposure dose of 200 or more rad had a significant relationship with lung cancer incidence, and the incidence was highest among the 20–29 age group. For histological type, the incidence of small cell carcinoma in the 100 or more rad exposed

TABLE IV.   Incidence of Lung Cancer by Radiation Dose, 1950–80
(Adjusted for City, Sex, and Age ATB)

Item	T65D in rad					
	Total	0(A)	1–49(B)	50–99(C)	100–199(D)	200+(E)
Observed	792	281	355	47	58	51
Expected		316.7	372.0	44.2	31.7	27.4
Person-years ($\times 10^3$)	2,046.7	807.6	975.2	108.4	80.7	74.8
Incidence rate ($\times 10^3$)		0.343	0.369	0.411	0.707	0.721
Relative risk		1.00	1.08	1.20	2.06	2.10

Test: A: D ***; A: E ***; Trend ***.   *** $p < 0.001$.

COLORECTAL CANCER AMONG ATOMIC BOMB SURVIVORS

Hirofumi NAKATSUKA[*1] and Haruo EZAKI[*2]

*Second Department of Surgery, Hiroshima University School of Medicine[*1] and Department of Clinical Studies, Radiation Effects Research Foundation[*2]*

Studies on autopsied and surgical cases of colorectal cancer in Hiroshima and Nagasaki atomic bomb (A-bomb) survivors have not shown a relationship to radiation.

In a recent epidemiologic study made on a fixed population at the Radiation Effects Research Foundation (RERF), the risk of colon cancer was found to increase significantly with increasing radiation dose in both Hiroshima and Nagasaki, and also in both males and females. The dose effect for the cities and sexes combined was especially pronounced for cancer of the sigmoid colon. The effect of radiation was found to vary by age at the time of the bomb (ATB) and the effect was remarkable among those under age 20 ATB. The risk of rectal cancer was not found to increase significantly with radiation and the distribution of histological types for cancer of either the colon or rectum was unrelated to radiation dose.

The effect of A-bomb exposure on the postoperative survival rate for colorectal cancer patients was studied. No difference by radiation dose could be demonstrated.

In Japan, the incidence of colorectal cancer, and of colon cancer in particular, has been increasing. Therefore, close attention should be paid to changes occurring in A-bomb survivors.

Experimental evidence suggests that intestinal tumors, especially malignant tumors, can be induced in mice by whole-body irradiation (*23, 27*). In man, the development of colorectal cancer following pelvic irradiation for benign disorders or cancer of the cervix and uterus has been reported (*3, 5, 24*). Also, a study of patients treated for ankylosing spondylitis by radiation showed an excess of deaths from cancer of the large intestine (*4*).

In atomic bomb (A-bomb) survivors, diarrhea and bloody stools were observed as clinical symptoms of acute radiation sickness, and inflammation and ulcerative lesions of the mucosa of the intestinal tract were found histopathologically (*15*). Therefore, it is suspected that the intestinal tract was subject to considerable damage by ionizing radiation.

According to a recent report (*12*) on the RERF Life Span Study (LSS) sample, a radiation effect has been observed for colon cancer but not for rectal cancer. However, only a few reports have been made concerning the occurrence of malignant tumors of the large bowel in A-bomb survivors.

[*1] Kasumi 1-2-3, Minami-ku, Hiroshima 734, Japan (中塚博文).
[*2] Hijiyama Park 5-2, Minami-ku, Hiroshima 732, Japan (江崎治夫).

In this paper, the reports made to date on colorectal cancer in A-bomb survivors are summarized, the effect of A-bomb radiation on the occurrence of colorectal cancer is reviewed, and data on the postoperative survival rate for colorectal cancer patients are included.

Colorectal Cancer in Autopsied Cases

Liebow *et al.* (*15*) reported that hemorrhage and ulceration occurred very frequently in the gastrointestinal tract of patients who died between the third and sixth weeks after the bombings. Further, ulcerative lesions of the intestine, especially of the colon, occurred often in those who died after the sixth week. However, reports have rarely been made on autopsied cases in relation to the occurrence of malignant tumors in the intestinal tract.

Yamamoto and Kato (*31*) reported on 94 cases of malignant tumor of the intestinal tract found among the autopsied cases in the Atomic Bomb Casualty Commission (ABCC) and the Japanese National Institute of Health (JNIH) fixed population during the period 1948–70. In that report, which dealt with the tumor site, age distribution, and histological type, no relationship with radiation dose was observed.

Colorectal Cancer in Surgical Cases

Regarding surgical cases of colorectal cancer in A-bomb survivors of Hiroshima, 32 cases of colon cancer were reported by Sato *et al.* (*25*) and 25 cases of rectal cancer by Miyoshi *et al.* (*19*). According to these reports, colorectal cancer in survivors was characterized by the predominance of cases in advanced age, relatively advanced stages, and a high proportion of local infiltration which rendered radical resection impossible. Recently, Nakatsuka *et al.* (*21*) analyzed the postoperative survival of 81 A-bomb survivors of Hiroshima who had undergone surgery for colorectal cancer during 1958–82; they found no statistically significant difference in the survival rate between these cases and those in 198 nonexposed persons in the same period.

Azuma *et al.* (*1*) conducted a clinical study on 119 cases of colorectal cancer in Nagasaki survivors and reported a high rate of second primary cancer in these survivors.

Because the number of cases was small and there were problems with respect to the selection of control groups, these reports have not been able to demonstrate definitively the features of colorectal cancer in the population of survivors.

Colorectal Cancer in the RERF LSS Sample

In 1950, ABCC-JNIH established a fixed sample of approximately 100,000 subjects consisting of A-bomb survivors and their controls in Hiroshima and Nagasaki (*10*), and RERF is continuing a long-term follow-up study of this sample. Colorectal cancer in this sample will be discussed.

According to Beebe *et al.* (*2*), an analysis of mortality for the period 1950–74 did not demonstrate any obvious radiation effect in either colon cancer or rectal cancer. A significant relationship between colon cancer and radiation dose was found only among Hiroshima females. Tumor Registry data for the period 1959–70 showed a statistically significant increasing trend in incidence of colon cancer with increasing dose in both

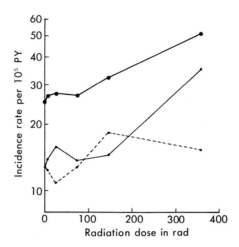

FIG. 1.   Colorectal cancer incidence rate by radiation dose and organ, Hiroshima and Nagasaki, 1950–80 (adjusted for age ATB, sex, and city). ●—●, colorectal*** (551 cases); •—•, colon*** (286 cases); •---•, rectum[NS] (test for linear trend; NS, $p>0.10$; *** $p<0.001$).

Hiroshima ($p<0.02$) and Nagasaki ($p<0.05$). However, the incompleteness of the Tumor Registry data and possible bias in identification of cases leave problems that need to be resolved. Subsequently, Kato and Schull (*12*) extended the study period to 1950–78, and reported a significant association between radiation dose and colon cancer mortality. An association between radiation dose and colon cancer incidence was also suggested by the analysis of Wakabayashi *et al.* (*28*) who used data from the Nagasaki Tumor Registry for the period 1959–78. However, in no study reported so far has there been observed any relationship between rectal cancer and A-bomb radiation.

Motivated by the results described above, Nakatsuka *et al.* (*22*) conducted a review of the relationship between exposure dose (tentative 1965 dose revised (T65DR)) (*13, 18*) and incidence of colorectal cancer. This study included a clinicopathological reexamination of cases in the LSS Extended Sample who were diagnosed as colorectal cancer based on the autopsy and surgical specimens of ABCC-RERF, Hiroshima and Nagasaki Tumor and Tissue Registry data, and death certificates for 1950–80.

According to this study, the incidence of colon cancer among A-bomb survivors increased significantly with radiation dose ($p<0.001$), but that of rectal cancer did not ($p>0.10$) (Fig. 1).

1. City and sex

These data showed a statistically significant increasing trend in the incidence of colon cancer with increasing dose in both Hiroshima ($p<0.001$) and Nagasaki ($p<0.05$) (Fig. 2). A dose response was also found for males ($p<0.01$) and for females ($p<0.001$) (Fig. 3).

2. Age at the time of the bomb (ATB)

The relative risk of colon cancer in the 100 or more rad dose group as compared to the 0 rad group differed by age ATB, being especially large for those exposed at age less than 20 (Table I).

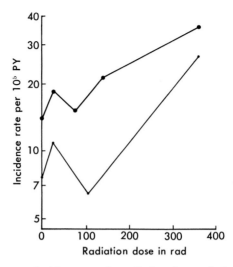

Fig. 2. Colon cancer incidence rate by radiation dose and city (adjusted for age ATB and sex). ●—●, Hiroshima*** (239 cases); •—•, Nagasaki* (47 cases) (test for linear trend; * $p<0.05$; *** $p<0.001$).

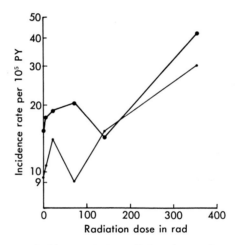

Fig. 3. Colon cancer incidence rate by radiation dose and sex (adjusted for age ATB and city). ●—●, male** (145 cases); •—•, female** (141 cases) (test for linear trend; ** $p<0.01$).

Table I. Relative Risk of Colon Cancer Incidence by Age ATB and Period (100+vs. 0 rad)

Period	Age ATB in years					
	Total	20	20–29	30–39	40–49	50+
Total	2.0**	4.5**	2.1	1.7	1.8[Sug.]	1.3
	(99,33)	(6,7)	(8,4)	(31,9)	(32,9)	(22,4)
1950–64	1.3	—	—	2.1	0	1.2
	(16,3)	(0,0)	(0,1)	(4,1)	(5,0)	(7,1)
1965–80	2.1**	5.3**	1.5	1.7	2.1*	1.5
	(83,30)	(6,7)	(8,3)	(27,8)	(27,9)	(15,3)

Numbers in parentheses are colon cancer cases in the 0 rad and 100+ rad groups, respectively.
Two-sample Mantel-Haenszel test: Suggestive, $p<0.10$; * $p<0.05$; ** $p<0.01$.

3. *Primary site of colon cancer*

A radiation effect was observed for cancer originating in each of the following sites: cecum plus ascending colon ($p<0.01$), transverse plus descending colon ($p<0.05$), and sigmoid colon ($p<0.001$). Among these sites, the dose-response effect was most remarkable in the sigmoid colon (Fig. 4).

4. *Histopathological type*

Cancer was classified by histological type according to the General Rules for Clinical and Pathological Studies on Cancer of Colon, Rectum, and Anus (*11*). Neither

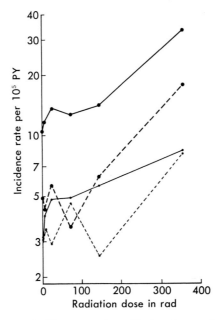

FIG. 4. Colon cancer incidence rate by radiation dose and site-confirmed cases (adjusted for age ATB, sex, and city). ●—●, colon*** (251 cases); ●---●, sigmoid*** (111 cases); •—•, cecum+ascending** (76 cases); •---•, transverse+descending* (64 cases) (test for linear trend; * $p<0.05$; ** $p<0.01$; *** $p<0.001$).

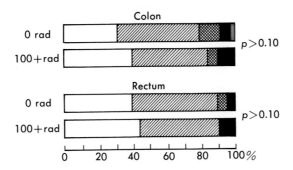

FIG. 5. Distribution of histological type of colorectal cancer by radiation dose. □, well differentiated adenocarcinoma; ▨, moderately differentiated adenocarcinoma; ▒, poorly differentiated adenocarcinoma; ■, mucinous carcinoma+signet ring cell carcinoma; ‖‖, other.

colon nor rectal cancer showed a significant difference in distribution of histopathological type between the 0 rad group and the 100 or more rad group (Fig. 5).

Survival of Colorectal Cancer Patients after Surgery

A study was made on the effects of A-bomb exposure on the postoperative survival rate for colorectal cancer patients (20).

Of the 730 cases, surgery was performed on 545 cases, of whom 148 cases who died within one month after surgery or whose records were missing were excluded from the analysis (Table II). Figure 6 shows the cumulative survival rates by type of surgery and cancer site.

For colon cancer the survival rate was highest for curative resection followed by noncurative resection and without resection. For rectum cancer, the survival rate of curative resection was the highest, followed by noncurative resection and without resection, the latter two being at almost the same level. The difference in the survival rates was found to be significant by the Mantel-Cox test (16).

TABLE II. Number of Operated Cases by Type of Operation and Cancer Site

Type of operation	Site			
	Total	Colon	Rectum	Unknown
Total	397	218	178	1
Curative resection[a]	238	134	103	1
Noncurative resection[a]	85	58	27	—
Without resection	62	22	40	—
Polypectomy	6	2	4	—
Unknown	6	2	4	—

Excluding operative deaths and cases whose stage of cancer, age, sex, and date of surgery are unknown.
[a] General Rules for Clinical and Pathological Studies on Cancer of Colon, Rectum, and Anus," 2nd ed., Japanese Research Society for Cancer of Colon and Rectum, 1980.

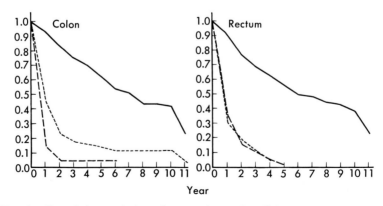

FIG. 6. Cumulative survival rate by type of operation. Colon: ——, curative resection (n=134); ----, non curative resection (n=58); — —, without resection (n=22); Mantel-Cox test, p<0.001. Rectum: ——, curative resection (n=103); ----, non curative resection (n=27); — —, without resection (n=40); Mantel-Cox test, p<0.001.

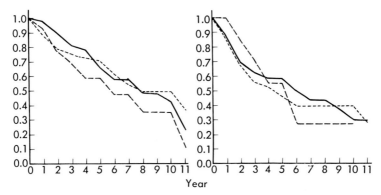

Year

Fig. 7. Cumulative survival rate by radiation dose. Colon: ——, 0 (n=39); - - - -, 1–99 (n=52); — —, 100+ (n=13); Mantel-Cox test, p>0.10. Rectum; ——, 0 (n= 33); - - - -, 1–99 (n=34); — —, 100+ (n=7); Mantel-Cox test, p>0.10.

The relationship between survival rate and radiation dose was examined for only cases of curative resection. Cases whose exposure dose was unknown and those who were not in the city ATB were excluded (Fig. 7). The survival rate of colon cancer cases tended to be slightly lower in the 100 or more rad group than in the other two groups. For rectum cancer, the survival rate for the 100 or more rad group was better than for the other groups during the early postoperative period, but the long-term survival rate of this group was found to be slightly lower. However, comparison of the survival curves of these groups by the Mantel-Cox test demonstrated no statistically significant difference.

As there are many factors which affect the postoperative survival rates, it is necessary to examine the effects of other factors in order to determine the effect of radiation. The potential factors are age at the time of operation, period of operation, sex, stage of cancer, and histopathological grade of cancer (Fig. 8). No difference could be observed by age, period of operation, and histopathological grade of cancer. By sex, the survival rates for both colon and rectum cancer cases were significantly higher in females. The survival rate of colon cancer cases was observed to be higher in Group A of Dukes' classification than in Groups B and C, but the difference was not statistically significant. The survival rate of rectum cancer cases was significantly higher in the order of A, B, and C.

It is necessary to take these factors into account in order to determine the effect of A-bomb exposure on the postoperative survival rate. For this purpose, classification into many groups with the same factors is necessary, but such classification makes the number of cases in each cell so small that comparison is not possible. By using Cox's proportional hazard model, which enables comparison of survival curves while taking into account the effects of many factors simultaneously, the regression coefficient of each group was examined, but no difference by radiation dose could be demonstrated in the postoperative survival rate for either colon or rectum cancer.

DISCUSSION

The occurrence of intestinal cancer due to radiation exposure has been confirmed by animal experiments (8, 23, 27). Malignant tumors have been noted to develop in humans

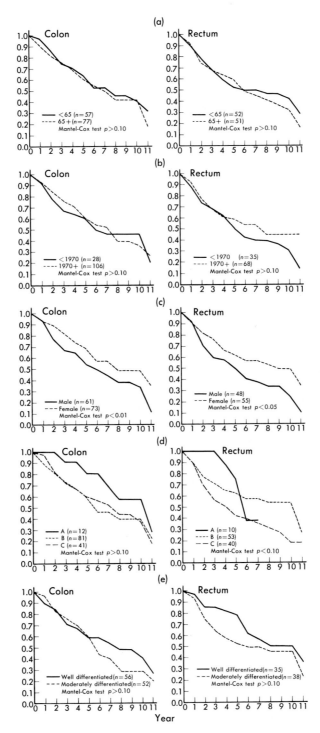

FIG. 8. Survival rate by age at operation (a), period at operation (b), sex (c), stage of cancer (Dukes' classification) (d), and histopathological grade (e).

following radiation therapy for lesions of the uterus or ovary (*3, 24*): tumors were found to originate in the part of the large bowel that lay in the irradiation field.

However, among epidemiological studies made so far on man, there have been few reports of a definite effect of radiation in the genesis of colorectal cancer.

In RERF studies on the LSS population, a significant relationship with ionizing radiation has been observed for colon cancer, but not for rectal cancer, and the radiation effect on the colon was remarkable for sigmoid colon. Such a difference in A-bomb radiation effect by site for colorectal cancer is of great interest, since it has been reported from epidemiological studies (*7, 29, 30*) that the colon is more susceptible than the rectum to carcinogenic effects of exogenous factors such as diet, and that this tendency is remarkable in the sigmoid colon.

In a comparison between Hiroshima and Nagasaki, a difference was observed in the incidence of leukemia (*9*), perhaps due to the difference of radiation quality. However, no obvious difference in the colon cancer dose-response relationship has been observed between the two cities (*22*). This problem should be studied further since the radiation dose estimates are currently being reassessed.

The effect of age ATB on the occurrence of malignant tumors is being studied in detail with regard to hormone-dependent tumors such as breast cancer (*26*) and thyroid cancer (*6*). Matsuura *et al.* (*17*) reported on stomach cancer, which, among digestive organ cancer, showed a remarkable elevation in incidence in those under age 30 ATB. On the other hand, Nakatsuka *et al.* (*22*) reported that they found an elevation in the incidence of colon cancer in those exposed to 100 or more rad who were under age 20 ATB, and that this group needs to be followed very carefully as it is now reaching the age when colon cancer is prone to develop.

The distribution of histological types shows no difference between the radiation dose groups. Castro *et al.* (*3*) reported that the percentage of mucinous carcinoma is high in cases exposed to medical radiation; however, the cases they reported were exposed to high partial-body doses of several thousand rad as therapy for cervical or uterine cancer. The A-bomb survivors, in contrast, are a general population exposed to an average of 27.2 rad (*12*).

The present report centers around studies which are based on a fixed population of A-bomb survivors, and which concern the effect of ionizing radiation on the occurrence of colorectal cancer. In recent years in Japan colorectal cancer, and colon cancer in particular, has shown a gradually increasing trend (*14, 29*) possibly due to westernization of diet and an increasing number of people of advanced age. Thus it remains imperative to pay attention to changes occurring in atomic bomb survivors.

REFERENCES

1. Azuma, K., Yamashita, I., Noda, S., Sakaeda, K., and Noguchi, K. Colorectal cancer in atomic bomb survivors in the Japanese Red Cross Nagasaki A-bomb Hospital. *Jpn. J. Gastroenterol. Surg.*, **14**, 869 (1981) (in Japanese).
2. Beebe, G. W., Kato, H., and Land, C. E. Life Span Study Report 8. Mortality experience of atomic bomb survivors, 1950–74. RERF Tech. Rep. 1-77 (1977).
3. Castro, E. B., Rosen, P. P., and Quan, S.H.Q. Carcinoma of large intestine in patients irradiated for carcinoma of cervix and uterus. *Cancer*, **31**, 45–52 (1973).
4. Court Brown, W. M. and Doll, R. Mortality from cancer and other causes after radiotherapy for ankylosing spondylitis. *Br. Med. J.*, **2**, 1327–1332 (1965).

5. Doll, R. and Smith, P. G. The long term effects of x-irradiation in patients treated for metropathia heamorrhagica. *Br. J. Radiol.*, **41**, 362–368 (1968).
6. Ezaki, H. Thyroid cancer occurring in Hiroshima atomic bomb survivors (1958–79). *J. Jpn. Pract. Surg. Soc.*, **44**, 1127–1137 (1983) (in Japanese).
7. Haenszel, W. and Correa, P. Cancer of the colon and rectum and adenomatous polyps; A review of epidemiologic findings. *Cancer*, **28**, 14–24 (1971).
8. Hirose, F., Fukazawa, K., Watanabe, H., Terada, Y., Fujii, I., and Otsuka, S. Induction of rectal carcinoma in mice by local x-irradiation. *Gann*, **68**, 669–680 (1977).
9. Ishimaru, T., Hoshino, T., Ichimaru, M., Okada, H., Tomiyasu, T., Tsuchimoto, T., and Yamamoto, T. Leukemia in atomic bomb survivors, Hiroshima and Nagasaki, 1 October 1950–30 September 1966. *Radiat. Res.*, **45**, 216–233 (1971).
10. Jablon, S., Ishida, M., and Beebe, G. W. JNIH-ABCC Life Span Study, Report 2 Motality in selection 1 and 2, October 1950—September 1959. *Radiat. Res.*, **21**, 423–445 (1964) (ABCC Tech. Rep. 1-63).
11. Japanese Research Society for Cancer of Colon and Rectum (ed). "General Rules for Clinical and Pathological Studies on Cancer of Colon, Rectum and Anus," The 2nd ed. (1980) Kanehara Publishing Company, Tokyo (in Japanese).
12. Kato, H. and Schull, W. J. Studies of mortality of A-bomb survivors. 7. Mortality, 1950–78: Part 1. Cancer mortality. *Radiat. Res.*, **90**, 395–432 (1982) (RERF Tech. Rep. 12-80).
13. Kerr, G. D. and Solomon, D. L. The epicenter of the Nagasaki weapon: A reanalysis of available data with recommended values. Oak Ridge National Laboratory, ORNL-TM-5139, U.S.A. (1979).
14. Lee, J.A.H. Recent trends of large bowel cancer in Japan compared to United States and England and Wales. *Int. J. Epidemiol.*, **5**, 187–194 (1976).
15. Liebow, A. A., Warren, S., and DeCoursey, E. Pathology of atomic bomb casualties. *Am. J. Pathol.*, **25**, 853–1029 (1949).
16. Mantel, N. Evaluation of survival data and the new rank order statistics arising in its consideration. *Cancer Chemother., Rep.*, **50**, 163–170 (1966).
17. Matsuura, H., Yamamoto, T., Sekine, I., Ochi, Y., and Otake, M. Pathological and epidemiologic study of gastric cancer in atomic bomb survivors, Hiroshima and Nagasaki, 1959–77. *Radiat. Res.*, **25**, 111–129 (1984).
18. Milton, R. C. and Shohoji, T. Tentative 1965 radiation dose estimation for atomic bomb survivors, Hiroshima and Nagasaki. ABCC Tech. Rep. 1-68 (1968).
19. Miyoshi, Y., Seto, Y., Morinaga, K., Yukata, H., Hirose, S., Sasaki, K., and Ogawa, Y. Surgical studies of rectal cancer at the Hiroshima Atomic Bomb Hospital for 10 years. *J. Hiroshima Med. Assoc.*, **33**, 313–315 (1980) (in Japanese).
20. Nakatsuka, H., Ezaki, H., and Shimizu, Y. Survival rate of colorectal cancer patients after surgery. In preparation.
21. Nakatsuka, H., Tamura, T., Nishiki, M., Kodama, M., and Ezaki, H. Review of colorectal cancer cases in atomic bomb survivors. *Abstr. Gen. Meet. Jpn. Pract. Surg. Soc.*, **44**, 486 (1983) (in Japanese).
22. Nakatsuka, H., Yamamoto, T., Shimizu, Y., Takahashi, M., Ezaki, H., Tahara, E., Sekine, I., Shimoyama, T., Mochinaga, N., Tomita, M., and Tsuchiya, R. Colorectal cancer among atomic bomb survivors in Hiroshima and Nagasaki (1950–80). Collection of lectures of 25th Late A-bomb Radiation Effect Research Meeting. *Nagasaki Med. J.*, **59**, 473–480 (1984) (in Japanese).
23. Nowell, P. C., Cole, L. J., and Ellis, M. E. Induction of intestinal carcinoma in the mouse by whole-body fast-neutron irradiation. *Cancer Res.*, **16**, 873–876 (1956).
24. Sandler, R. S. and Sandler, D. P. Radiation-induced cancer of the colon and rectum: Assessing the risk. *Gastroenterology*, **84**, 51–57 (1983).
25. Sato, M., Yo, S., Sasao, T., Sasaki, K., and Ogawa, Y. Surgical studies of colon cancer at

the Hiroshima Atomic Bomb Hospital for 10 years. *Nagasaki Med. J.*, **53**, 398–403 (1978) (in Japanese).

26. Tokunaga, M., Norman, J., Asano, M., Tokuoka, S., Ezaki, H., Nishimori, I., and Tsuji Y. Malignant breast tumors among atomic bomb survivors, Hiroshima and Nagasaki, 1950–74. *J. Natl. Cancer Inst.*, **62**, 1347–1359 (1979) (RERF Tech. Rep. 17-77).

27. Upton, A. C., Kimball, A. W., Furth, J., Christenbery, K. W., and Benedict, W. H. Some delayed effects of atomic bomb radiation in mice. *Cancer Res.*, **20**, 1–60 (1960).

28. Wakabayashi, T., Kato, H., Ikeda, T., and Schull, W. Life Span Study Report 9, part 3, Tumor Registry data, Nagasaki 1959–78. RERF Tech. Rep. 6-81 (1981).

29. Watanabe, Y., Kawamoto, K., Kajiwara, Y., Akasaka, Y., and Kawai, K. Epidemiological study on cancer of the large intestine in Japan (1) Fundamental analysis from mortality of the large intestine in Japan. *J. Jpn. Soc. Colo-proctol.*, **36**, 607–614 (1983) (in Japanese).

30. Wynder, E. L. The epidemiology of large bowel cancer. *Cancer Res.*, **35**, 3388–3394 (1975).

31. Yamamoto, T., and Kato, H. Malignant tumors of the intestines found in a fixed population of Hiroshima. *Proc. Jpn. Cancer Assoc.*, **30**, 112 (1971).

BREAST CANCER IN ATOMIC BOMB SURVIVORS

Masayoshi Tokunaga,[*1,*2] Shoji Tokuoka,[*3] and
Charles E. Land[*4]

*Department of Pathology, Kagoshima Municipal Hospital,[*1] Department of
Pathology and Department of Epidemiology and Statistics, Radiation
Effects Research Foundation,[*2] Second Department of Pathology,
Faculty of Medicine, Hiroshima University,[*3] and Radiation
Epidemiology Branch, National Cancer Institute, NIH[*4]*

Thirty eight years after the atomic bombings, studies of the Radiation Effects Research Foundation (RERF) on the extended Life Span
Study (LSS) sample have continued to provide important information on
radiation carcinogenesis. The third breast cancer survey among this sample revealed 564 cases during the period 1950–80, of which 412 were reviewed microscopically. The following statements reflect the conclusions
from the current investigation; 1) the relationship between radiation dose
and breast cancer incidence was consistent with linearity and did not differ
markedly between the Hiroshima and Nagasaki survivors, 2) a dose-related breast cancer risk was observed among women who were in their
first decade of life at the time of exposure, 3) the relative risk of radiation-
induced breast cancer decreased with increasing age at exposure, 4) the
pattern over time of age-specific breast cancer incidence is similar for exposed and control women (that is, exposed women have more breast
cancer than control women but the excess risk closely follows normal risk
as expressed by age-specific population rates), and 5) radiation-induced
breast cancer appears to be morphologically similar to other breast cancer.

There is general agreement that ionizing radiation is one of the best understood
and most thoroughly studied environmental carcinogens and that female breast cancer
may be the best understood site of radiation-induced cancer in humans.

In 1965, Mackenzie (*13*) reported an increased risk of breast cancer for women who
received repeated fluoroscopy during pneumothorax treatment for tuberculosis in a Nova
Scotia sanatorium. At that time, he found 13 cases of breast cancer in 271 patients subjected to repeated chest fluoroscopy as compared with only one case which developed
in 570 patients who were not fluoroscoped. This study group was later extended by
Myrden and Hiltz (*17*).

Boice and Monson (*5*) studied 1,047 women treated in Massachusetts tuberculosis
sanatoria by pneumothorax who received an average of 102 chest fluoroscopies during
1935–54, and a control group of 717 nonexposed tuberculosis patients. Many of the
patients had been treated as teenagers, in contrast to the Nova Scotia series in which

---

[*1] Kajiya-cho 20-17, Kagoshima 892 and [*2] Hijiyama Park 5-2, Minami-ku, Hiroshima 730, Japan
(德永正義).
[*3] Kasumi 1-2-3, Minami-ku, Hiroshima 734, Japan (德岡昭治).
[*4] Landow Building, Room 3A22, Bethesda, Maryland 20892, U.S.A.

patients were appreciably older when treated. Individual dosimetry yielded an estimated average breast tissue dose of 150 rad in 100 exposures, averaging 1.5 rad per exposure. Breast cancer incidence was high among the exposed (41 observed *vs.* 23.5 expected according to population rates), and the excess was proportional to dose. The excess risk was estimated as 6.2 breast cancer cases per million women per year per rad. The minimal appearance time for radiogenic breast cancer was estimated to be 10 to 15 years, while the risk extended for as long as 40 years after exposure. The Massachusetts data were interpreted as suggesting that early adult life is a time when the breast is particularly susceptible to cancer induction, that proliferating tissue may be sensitive to irradiation, and that multiple low-dose exposures cumulated over many years may be as effective in inducing breast cancer as less fractionated, or even single, exposures (*2, 5*).

Radiation induced breast cancer was observed among women with histories of X-ray therapy for acute postpartum mastitis by the studies of Mettler *et al.* (*15*) and Shore *et al.* (*18*). Shore *et al.* (*18*) found 36 (6.3%) breast cancer cases in 571 women treated with X-rays for acute postpartum mastitis compared with 32 (3.2%) in 933 nonirradiated siblings and patients treated by other means. The mean cumulative dose to both breasts was 247 rad, and the overall excess risk of breast cancer was about 8–10 cases per million women per year per rad. Women over age 30 years at radiation treatment had as great an excess risk of breast cancer as did younger women. A linear dose response was observed, and the relatively minor fractionation of exposure (1–5 fractions) did not appear to reduce carcinogenic action.

Baral *et al.* (*1*) reported a study of women given radiation therapy for benign breast disorders in Sweden, and found young women to be at greatest radiation risk; generally risk decreased with age at exposure.

In addition to these breast cancer studies among medically exposed populations, continuing follow-up studies of breast cancer incidence among female survivors of the Hiroshima and Nagasaki atomic bomb (A-bomb) explosions provided important knowledge about radiation breast carcinogenesis. In 1967, Wanebo *et al.* (*24*) studied 31 cases of breast cancer (27 with histological diagnoses) occurring among examined members of the Atomic Bomb Casualty Commission (ABCC) Adult Health Study (AHS) sample of A-bomb survivors in Hiroshima and Nagasaki for the period 1958–66. Of the 18 histologically verified cases occurring among exposed women examined at least once during the period 1958–66, and for whom dose estimates could be made, 50% had dose estimates of 90 rad or more as compared to only 24% expected by chance alone.

In 1974, McGregor *et al.* (*14*) studied breast cancer incidence among members of the much larger ABCC Life Span Study (LSS) sample for the period 1950–69. In this study, 231 breast cancer cases were identified among 63,275 female A-bomb survivors and nonexposed controls and 187 were among survivors for whom dose estimates were available. The estimated absolute risk per rad was 1.9 excess cases per 10^6 person-years at risk. The data suggested that the breast tissue of adolescent females, as compared to older women, was especially sensitive to the effects of ionizing radiation.

The similarity observed by McGregor *et al.* (*14*) between the two cities was interesting partly because baseline (that is, nonradiogenic) breast cancer rates in Nagasaki have historically been only about half those in Hiroshima, but mainly because the radiation from the Hiroshima bomb was for a long time believed to contain a substantial neutron component absent in the radiation from the Nagasaki bomb. Neutrons generally are more damaging than gamma rays, and indeed, excess risk for cancer other than breast cancer has tended to be greater in Hiroshima than in Nagasaki. Approximate equality of the excess risk per unit dose between the two cities was interpreted as suggesting approximate equivalence of gamma ray and neutron radiation for the induction of breast cancer. More recent dosimetric studies suggest that the quality of the radiation received from the two bombs was not so different after all; reassessment of dosimetry is now underway, and for the present it is difficult to evaluate this aspect of the breast cancer data from Hiroshima and Nagasaki.

The second incidence study among the extended LSS sample was performed by Tokunaga *et al.* (*22*) and increased the number of cases to 360 during 1950–74. This incidence survey found similar dose-incidence relationships, both consistent with linearity, in Hiroshima and Nagasaki. Age at exposure was an important biological modifier of risk, with the greatest relative and absolute increase occurring among those 10 to 19 years at the time of the bomb (ATB). No excess risk was observed among those exposed under age 10 ATB, although it was recognized that these women might not yet be old enough for a risk to be detected. A rather peculiar relationship was observed among those 40 to 49 ATB in that no radiation related risk was detected, and as dose increased, the incidence of breast cancer actually decreased.

Summary of Findings Prior to the Third LSS Survey

The nearly simultaneous publications in 1979 of epidemiological studies of breast cancer risk in three different irradiated populations, the Boice-Monson study (*5*) of Massachusetts tuberculosis patients with multiple chest fluoroscopies, the Shore *et al.* (*18*) survey of patients given X-ray therapy for benign breast disease in Rochester, New York, and the second ABCC-RERF (1950–74) study (*22*) based on the extended LSS sample of A-bomb survivors in Hiroshima and Nagasaki prompted a reanalysis in parallel of the basic data from all three studies (*4, 10*). The central feature of this reanalysis was that, in so far as possible, the data were identically subdivided by age at exposure, and risk was observed for closely similar periods following exposure. For similar exposure ages, risk estimates obtained by linear regression of risk on radiation dose were closely similar for the three data sets, despite differences in underlying population rates, fractionation of exposure, and the extent to which irradiation extended to parts of the body other than the breast (Fig. 1). These differences were substantial, including a five-fold difference between Japanese and American population rates, a single exposure among the A-bomb survivors *vs.* 1–19 fractions among the Rochester patients and 100 or more fractions among the Massachusetts tuberculosis patients, and whole-body A-bomb exposure *vs.* chest irradiation from fluoroscopy *vs.* therapeutic X-ray limited to one or two breasts. For all three data sets the observed dose response appeared linear, a finding that is consistent with the lack of a dose fractionation effect. Other important characteristics of the three data sets were, first, that excess risk did not appear until ages of normally appreciable breast cancer risk, regardless of age at exposure, and that after it appeared the temporal patterns of excess and background risk were closely similar. Second, at ages of normally appreciable risk, the excess following exposure at ages 10–19 was markedly higher than that following exposure at older age.

The observation that multiple low-dose exposures did not produce significantly less cancer per unit dose than less highly fractionated exposures suggests that radiation damage is cumulative and that highly fractionated X-irradiation may be as effective in

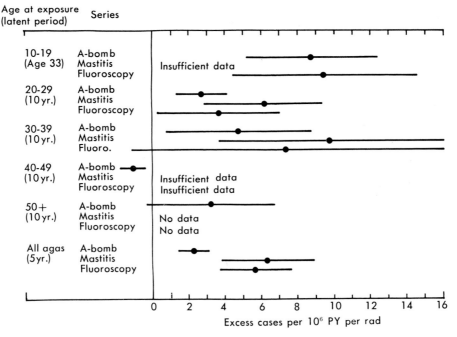

FIG. 1. Excess breast cancer risk per rad with 90% confidence intervals: parallel and analysis of three exposed populations.

inducing breast cancer as single or less fractionated exposures. The interpretation of these results is of particular public health importance, since the radiation of usual medical examination, cancer screening, or therapy is received from repeated exposure to low dose.

The Third LSS Follow-up Survey

As in the two earlier surveys of breast cancer incidence in the LSS extended sample (14, 22), an attempt was made to ascertain all diagnoses of breast cancer obtainable from resources available locally in Hiroshima and Nagasaki. The most wide-ranging of these resources is the system by which death certificate diagnoses routinely are made available to RERF from death certificates filed anywhere in Japan for members of the LSS sample. All death certificates for 1950–80 with breast cancer listed as either the underlying cause, a complication, or a contributing condition were included in the initial ascertainment. Information was collected from the series of indexed cases in the RERF autopsy program, the RERF collection of surgical specimens, the Tumor Registries maintained since 1959 and the Tissue Registries maintained since 1971 by the City and Prefectural Medical Associations of Hiroshima and Nagasaki, the records of the medical schools of Hiroshima and Nagasaki Universities, and records of more than 50 hospitals in both cities.

A total of 564 breast cancer cases was identified for the period 1950–80 among the 63,300 women in the extended LSS sample, which includes nearly all residents of Hiroshima and Nagasaki in 1950 who had been exposed within 2,500 m from ground zero, 15,400 nonexposed women who migrated or returned to the cities after August 1945, and an age-matched sample of women exposed between 2,500–10,000 m from ground zero.

1. Histological classification

Of the total of 564 female cases finally selected, 412 were accepted on the basis of pathology review. Of these, 301 cases were included in a review by a binational panel of pathologists from Japan and the United States on the basis of an incomplete ascertainment of cases through 1978 (*23*). The distribution of histological types in exposed and nonexposed groups is presented in Table I for the 412 cancer cases reviewed histologically by the investigators. According to contingency table analysis there was no evidence that the histological type is related to city, age ATB, age at diagnosis, calender time, radiation dose, or any combination of these factors. In particular, there was no tendency for one or more histological types or subtypes to characterize radiation-induced breast cancer. Although there have been no reported pathological studies of breast cancer among medically exposed populations, the present results provide strong evidence that radiation induced breast cancer appears to be morphologically similar to other breast cancer. One interpretation of these results is that the histological type of breast cancer is influenced by other factors but not by whether or not radiation is one initiator.

2. Linear dose response

The most important finding of the studies to date is that of linearity of the dose response for radiation-induced breast cancer, together with the similar pattern of risk for the two cities (Fig. 2). Linear regressions of age-standardized rates on total (gamma ray plus neutron) tentative 1965 dose (T65D) to breast tissue gave estimates of 4.0 ± 0.7 and 3.0 ± 0.7 excess cases per million women per year per rad for Hiroshima and Nagasaki,

TABLE I.   Distribution of Histological Type of Breast Cancer by Dose

Histological type	T65D in rad							
	NIC[c]	0–9	10–49	50–99	100–199	200+	Unknown	Total
Noninvasive[a]	4	6	—	1	—	2	—	13
Invasive								
a. Ductal								
0. CSF[b]	8	17	2	4	3	10	1	45
1. Papillotubular	5	7	4	—	0	2	2	20
2. Medullary tubular	14	24	9	7	2	7	4	67
3. Scirrhous	31	91	27	4	16	14	3	186
b. Predominant ductal component	7	21	9	2	3	3	—	45
c. Lobular	—	1	1	1	2	—	—	5
d. Mucinous	—	7	—	—	—	2	—	9
e. Medullary	1	3	—	—	—	—	—	4
f. Tubular	—	—	0	2	—	—	—	2
g. Secretory	—	1	—	—	—	1	—	2
h. Apocrine	—	1	—	—	—	—	—	1
i. Carcinoma with metaplasia	—	—	—	—	—	1	—	1
j. Paget's Disease								
0. *In situ* only	1	1	2	—	—	—	—	4
1. With invasive carcinoma	—	0	2	—	1	—	—	3
k. Other	2	3	—	—	—	—	—	5
Total	73	183	56	21	27	42	10	412

[a] All noninvasive carcinomas were intraductal; there were no lobular carcinomas *in situ*.

[b] Cannot subclassify further.

[c] Not in the city.

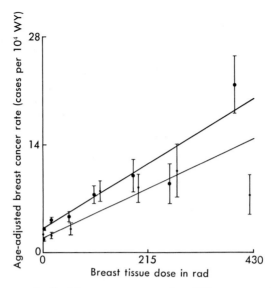

FIG. 2. Age-standardized breast cancer rates (case/10⁴ women-year) by estimated
dose to breast tissue, Hiroshima (●) and Nagasaki (•), 1950–80.

respectively. The difference between the two cities is not statistically significant. The
result of a linear dose response is approximately similar to that of the previous studies
(*14, 22*) and of the studies of populations medically exposed (*5, 18*).

3. Bilateral breast cancer

There were ten bilateral cases in the series, of which seven were from Hiroshima
and three from Nagasaki. All were among women under age 35 ATB; the proportion of
cases with bilateral cancer decreased with increasing age ATB. There were two bilateral
cases with over 300 rad kerma and one for whom no exposure estimate could be calculated;
two cases were nonexposed, and the rest had estimated kerma values under 5 rad. The
dose distribution of the nine cases with estimates showed that the incidence of bilateral
breast cancer increased with increasing dose, but not disproportionally when compared
with unilateral cancer (Table II).

4. Age at exposure

One of the most significant findings for breast cancer, which concerns the temporal
pattern after exposure, is the age at exposure. Previous studies (*14, 22*) including the second
survey of the LSS sample provided strong evidence for cancer induction in females

TABLE II.   Incidence of Bilateral Breast Cancer by Dose, Adjusted for City and Age ATB

Item	T65D in rad							
	0[a]	1–9	10–49	50–99	100–199	200–299	300–399	400+
Women year (×100)	8,778	3,476	2,368	6,656	466	209	98	120
Observed	5	2	0	0	0	0	2	0
Expected	4.76	2.00	1.34	0.39	0.25	0.11	0.07	0.08
Relative risk	1.00	0.95	0	0	0	0	26.97	0

[a] 0 exposure group includes women who were not in either city ATB and 0 dose groups.

exposed at ages 10–39, with girls 10–19 years of age having the greatest risk. These results, that the radiation exposures between the ages of 10 and 19 years produce more breast cancer than do equivalent exposures at later ages, observed in two different populations (5, 22), have been incorporated into general models of breast carcinogenesis (3).

Moolgavkar et al. (16) have elaborated upon a two-stage model for breast carcinogenesis. The model assumes that two discrete and irreversible events are required for cell transformation. Since each event must occur during cell division, tissue growth and rapid cell turnover would influence susceptibility. Observations that the absence of a radiation effect in women exposed under age 10 is due to few cells dividing before the time of breast development (i.e., there are few susceptible cells at risk) were incorporated into the model.

This model was strongly influenced by the fact that radiation-associated risk is highest at puberty and falls with increasing age at irradiation, a finding consistent with a proliferative advantage of intermediate cells, in which one of the two irreversible events

TABLE III. Breast Cancer in the LSS Sample by Radiation Exposure and Age ATB, 1950–80.

| Age ATB | Item | T65D in rad | | | | | | Total[b] — | p value for trend |
		0[a] (0)[c]	1–9 (2.6)	10–49 (16.8)	50–99 (54.6)	100–199 (110.3)	200+ (271.0)		
0–9	Observed	6	5	5	5	2	1	24	0.02
	Expected	13.2	5.5	3.6	0.8	0.5	0.5		
	O/E	0.5	0.9	1.4	5.9	4.1	2.2		
	RR[d]	1.0	2.0	3.1	13.0	9.0	4.8		
10–19	Observed	55	18	22	9	13	24	141	<0.00001
	Expected	78.6	28.4	18.2	5.7	5.4	4.8		
	O/E	0.7	0.6	1.2	1.6	2.4	5.0		
	RR	1.0	0.9	1.7	2.3	3.4	7.2		
20–29	Observed	58	20	21	7	8	13	127	<0.00001
	Expected	69.7	26.7	17.8	5.3	3.7	3.8		
	O/E	0.8	0.8	1.2	1.3	2.1	3.4		
	RR	1.0	0.9	1.4	1.6	2.6	4.1		
30–39	Observed	60	24	11	4	7	10	116	<0.00001
	Expected	65.0	23.9	17.6	4.7	2.6	2.2		
	O/E	0.9	1.0	0.6	0.9	2.7	4.5		
	RR	1.0	1.1	0.7	0.9	3.0	4.9		
40–49	Observed	53	15	20	1	2	3	94	0.31
	Expected	52.7	18.4	14.7	4.0	2.4	1.9		
	O/E	1.0	0.8	1.4	0.3	0.8	1.6		
	RR	1.0	0.8	1.4	0.2	0.8	1.6		
50+	Observed	26	10	8	1	3	1	49	0.15
	Expected	27.0	10.7	7.7	2.0	0.9	0.7		
	O/E	1.0	0.9	1.0	0.5	3.4	1.4		
	RR	1.0	1.0	1.1	0.5	3.5	1.5		
Total	Observed	258	92	87	27	35	52	551	<0.000001
	Expected	306.3	113.6	79.4	22.5	15.4	13.8		
	O/E	0.8	0.8	1.1	1.2	2.3	3.8		
	RR	1.0	1.0	1.3	1.4	2.7	4.5		

[a] 0 exposure group includes NIC and 0 dose groups.
[b] Total excludes survivors with unknown dose.
[c] Average tissue dose in rad in parentheses.
[d] Relative risk.

has already occurred. This proliferative advantage would be greatly reduced at menopause when a decrease in the turnover rate of breast epithelium is accompanied by involution and dysfunction.

The estrogen window theory of Korenman (9) is concerned with the protective effect of progesterone on susceptibility to environmental carcinogens. According to this model, there are two main induction periods in a woman's life that are characterized by increased estrogen and diminished progesterone secretion. The hypothesis assumes that breast tissue is particularly susceptible to environmental carcinogens when these "endocrine windows" are open. This author noted that there are many observations consistent with this model such as the lack of a breast cancer excess in survivors exposed under age 10, the increased susceptibility of the radiation breast carcinogenesis exposed just before and around menarche and the concordance of the patterns of age specific incidence curves between exposed and nonexposed Japanese women.

The observations of the third LSS sample study (19–21) resulted in a new understanding concerning age at exposure. The recent data indicate that a dose related excess breast cancer risk was found among women who were in their first decade of life ATB (Table III). The distribution of the 24 cases from the sample under age 10 ATB and the expected distribution in the absence of a dose relationship are given below by estimated radiation dose. The data suggest a breast cancer risk among women exposed to 50 or more rad, that is, over seven times as high as that among women with less than 10 rad exposure, in relative terms a higher risk than has been observed in any older group. A test for linearly increasing trend in risk with increasing dose yields a one-tailed p value of 0.023. The second study of the LSS sample was based on a too short follow-up to reveal the radiation effect for women exposed at such young ages. The number of cases is still small, but nevertheless sufficient for statistical significance at the 5% level, even after correction for skewness of the LSS sample dose distribution. The age-specific dose response data summarized in Fig. 3 show an overall pattern of a decreasing trend in excess risk with increasing age ATB. Similar results, that persons exposed at younger ages tend to be at greater risk than those exposed later, have been observed in other studies

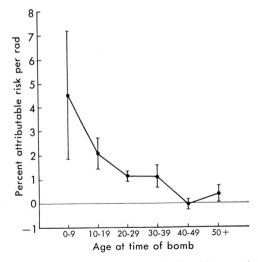

FIG. 3.   Linear regression estimates of excess relative risk per rad to breast tissue, by age ATB.

(7, 8). These data suggest that there are more cells susceptible to cancer induction in early life than later. It is also recommended to follow-up the entire postexposure life span to make clear the full picture of the mechanisms of radiation carcinogenesis.

Since the preliminary report (21) about the risk observed in the youngest group of the LSS sample, there have been three reports (6, 11, 12) of breast cancer among populations medically exposed before puberty. Hildreth et al. (6) found a 5.3-fold increased risk of breast cancer (95% confidence limits 1.6–17.4) among 2,872 individuals who received X-ray treatment in infancy (about 90% of them were less than six months of age at exposure) for an enlarged thymic gland as compared to 5,055 nonirradiated siblings. Li et al. (11) and Li and Rosen (12) found 7 breast cancer patients among 910 survivors of childhood cancer who received thoracic radiation therapy. These reports, together with those of the third LSS follow-up study, support the idea that radiation exposure before puberty may result in an increased risk of breast cancer later in life. The excess risk, however, does not seem to appear until ages normally associated with increased incidence.

Because these new findings are contrary to current theories (9, 16) on breast carcinogenesis, modification or reconsideration of these theories is necessary.

Summary of the Population Study Results of Radiation Breast Carcinogenesis

Opportunities for epidemiological studies of irradiated human populations have been pursued and much has been learned about radiation carcinogenesis. This new information will provide clues to evaluating biologic mechanisms of cancer causation. Large-scale studies have found dose-dependent increases in breast cancer incidence.

A)   In women with pulmonary tuberculosis whose artificial pneumothorax treatment was monitored by fluoroscopic chest examination (5).

B)   In women treated therapeutically with X-ray for acute postpartum mastitis (18) and for benign disease (1).

C)   In women treated therapeutically with irradiation in infancy for thymic enlargement (6) and for childhood tumors (11, 12).

D)   In Japanese women exposed to the A-bomb (14, 19, 22).

The results to date of these studies indicate that:

1.   The underlying relationship between radiation dose and breast cancer incidence is consistent with linearity (A, B, D), even at doses less than 50 rad (D).

2.   The relationship between radiation and breast cancer incidence may not differ markedly by radiation quality (D), although this inference is based on T65 dosimetry which will soon be replaced by one based on new calculations of bomb yield, energy spectrum, and attenuation by distance, shielding materials, and tissue.

3.   Age at exposure is an important biologic modifier of risk (A, B, C, D) with the greatest relative and absolute risk at young exposure ages (C, D), possibly even during infancy (C). The risk of radiation-induced breast cancer decreases with increasing age at exposure (A, B, D) with little or no dose-related excess risk in women irradiated over age 40 (D).

4.   The patterns of age-specific incidence of breast cancer are similar for exposed and nonexposed women (A, B, D); that is, exposed women have more breast cancer than nonexposed women, but the excess risk closely follows normal risk as expressed by age-specific population rates.

5.   The radiogenic cancer does not begin until the age of normally increased breast

cancer risk in nonexposed women (A, B, C, D); thus the induction period appears to be determined by events after exposure.

6. Excess risk may continue throughout life.

7. Fractionation of exposure does not appear to diminish risk (A, B).

8. Radiation-induced breast cancer appears to be morphologically similar to other breast cancer (D).

9. The incidence of bilateral cancer increases with increasing dose.

Acknowledgments

This manuscript is mainly based on the recent study entitled "Incidence of female breast cancer among atomic bomb survivors, Hiroshima and Nagasaki, 1950–80" performed at RERF (Research Protocol 17–81) with funding from the US National Cancer Institute (N0l-CP-01012).

We are indebted to the collaborators: Drs. Tsutomu Yamamoto, Masahide Asano, Haruo Ezaki, and Issei Nishimori.

The authors wish to thank the doctors of both cities who gave permission to use case information, and particularly the Tumor Registries of the Hiroshima and Nagasaki City Medical Associations, the Tissue Registries of the Hiroshima Prefectural Medical Association and Nagasaki City Medical Association, Hiroshima University School of Medicine, the Research Institute for Nuclear Medicine and Biology of Hiroshima University, Nagasaki University School of Medicine, the Atomic Disease Institute of Nagasaki University School of Medicine, and major hospitals of both cities.

REFERENCES

1. Baral, E., Larsson, L. E., and Mattson, B. Breast cancer following irradiation of the breast. *Cancer*, **40**, 2905–2910 (1977).

2. Boice, J. D., Jr. Multiple chest fluoroscopies and the risk of breast cancer. *In* "Advances in Medical Oncology, Research and Education, Vol. 1, Carcinogenesis," ed. G. P. Margison, pp. 147–156 (1979). Pergamon Press, Oxford and New York.

3. Boice, J. D., Jr. and Hoover, R. N. Radiogenic breast cancer: Age effects and implications for models of human carcinogenesis. *In* "Cancer: Achievements, Challenges, and Prospects for the 1980s," ed. J. H. Burchenal and H. F. Oettgen, Vol. 1, pp. 209–221 (1981). Grune & Stratton, New York.

4. Boice, J. D., Jr., Land, C. E., Shore, R. E., Norman, J. E., and Tokunaga, M. Risk of breast cancer following low-dose radiation exposure. *Radiology*, **132**, 589–597 (1979).

5. Boice, J. D., Jr. and Monson, R. R. Breast cancer in women after repeated fluoroscopic examinations of the chest. *J. Natl. Cancer Inst.*, **59**, 823–832 (1977).

6. Hildreth, N. G., Shore, R. E., and Hempelmann, L. H. Risk of breast cancer among women receiving radiation treatment in infancy for thymic enlargement. *Lancet*, **ii**, 273 (1983).

7. Ishimaru, T., Ezaki, H., Asano, M., Yagawa, K., Fujikura, T., Hayashi, Y., Nishida, T., Yasuda, K., Izumi, M., and Sato, K. Incidence of thyroid cancer among atomic bomb survivors and controls, Hiroshima and Nagasaki, 1958–79: Relationship to radiation absorbed dose in the thyroid. RERF Tech. Rep., in press.

8. Kato, H., and Schull, W. J. Studies of the mortality of A-bomb survivors. 7. Mortality 1950–1978. Part I. Cancer mortality. *Radiat. Res.*, **90**, 395–432 (1982).

9. Korenman, S. G. Oestrogen window hypothesis of the aetiology of breast cancer. *Lancet*, **i**, 700–701 (1980).

10. Land, C. E., Boice, J. D., Jr., Shore, R. E., Norman, J. E., and Tokunaga, M. Breast cancer risk from low-dose exposures to ionizing radiation: Results of parallel analysis of

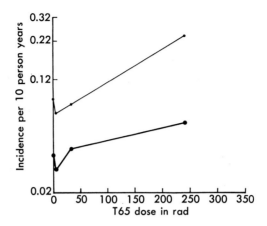

FIG. 2. Incidence of ovarian cancer by exposure dose and study period, Hiroshima and Nagasaki (microscopically reviewed cases). ●, 1950–64 ($p>0.10$); •, 1965–80 ($p<0.01$).

TABLE II. Relative Risk (100+ rad *vs.* 0 rad) of Ovarian Cancer Incidence by Age ATB

Method of ascertainment	Total	Age ATB in years				
		<20	20–29	30–39	40–49	50+
Total	2.2	5.0	2.1	1.5	1.5	0.95
	(74,19)	(9,7)	(14,5)	(18,3)	(18,3)	(15,1)
Histologically reviewed cases	1.9	4.4	2.5	1.1	1.9	—
	(51,12)	(6,4)	(10,4)	(16,2)	(9,2)	(10,0)

The numbers in parentheses are the number of cases in the 0 rad and 100+ rad groups, respectively.

TABLE III. Mean Time in Years from 1950 (Beginning of Follow-up) to Onset of Ovarian Cancer—All Cases

Age ATB in years	Total	T65 dose in rad				
		0	1–99	100+	Unknown	NIC[a]
Total	17.6±0.6	17.8±1.0	17.4±1.1	19.3±1.5	19.2±11.1	16.5±1.1
<20	21.8±1.2	26.2±0.9	25.3±1.1	21.3±1.3		17.1±2.8
20–39	18.9±0.9	20.2±1.3	17.5±1.9	19.6±3.1	19.2±11.1	17.8±1.7
40+	14.5±0.8	13.2±1.4	15.7±1.5	15.3±2.8		14.9±1.5

[a] Not in city ATB.

of time from exposure to the time of study commencement, to the average time for tumor development determined from the LSS (Table III).

In this regard, it was found that the latent period was not affected by the magnitude of exposure dose, but that it was inversely related to age ATB in all dose groups. For example, in the 100 or more rad group, the latent period was 15.3±2.8 years (the shortest) in the age group 40 and over ATB, 19.6±3.1 years in the age group 20–29 ATB, and 21.3±1.3 years (the longest) in the age group less than 20 ATB. This suggests that, as with breast cancer (*25*), ovarian cancer in A-bomb survivors does not develop until the host reaches an age normally associated with increased incidence, irrespective of either

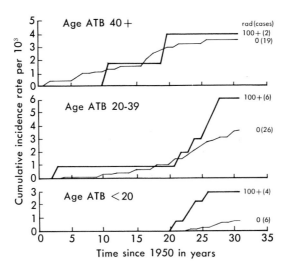

FIG. 3. Cumulative incidence rate (per 1,000) by exposure dose and ATB, Hiroshima and Nagasaki (microscopically reviewed cases).

age ATB or exposure dose; moreover, the latent period until tumor development is unrelated to exposure dose. Note, however, that in the age group less than 20 ATB, the mean latent period in the 100 or more rad exposure group was 21.3 ± 1.3 years, which appears to be significantly shorter than 26.2 ± 0.9 years in the 0 rad group; although the number of cases is quite small. The age group less than 20 ATB includes many individuals who had not reached the cancer age at the time of this study; this will necessitate further follow-up studies.

The cumulative incidence rate of ovarian cancer per 1,000 persons for the total 31 year period (1950–80) is shown in Fig. 3, stratified by the two exposure groups (100 or more rad *vs.* 0 rad) and three age ATB groups. An excess in the incidence rate for the 100 or more rad group *vs.* that for the 0 rad group was observed 10–15 years after 1950 (*i.e.*, 15–20 years after exposure) for the age 40 or more ATB group. For the age less than 20 ATB group, an excess in the incidence rate apparently comes later, around 25 years after exposure.

The finding also suggests that the minimum latent period for radiation induced ovarian cancer would be around 15–20 years, and the latent period is inversely related to age ATB.

The distribution of the 128 microscopically reviewed cases of ovarian cancer by histological type is shown in Table IV. Of the 128 cases 121 (94.5%) were carcinomas that belong to the WHO (*20*) category "Common Epithelial Tumors" (I). Of the remaining seven cases, four were granulosa cell tumors of "Sex Cord Stromal Tumors" category (II), two were teratomas associated with malignant transformation, and one was carcinoid, belonging to the "Germ Cell Tumors" category (IV).

The histological distribution in the 79 combined nonexposed and 0 rad group cases was 73 (92.4%), 3 (3.8%), and 3 (3.8%) in categories I, II, and IV, respectively. Because of differing criteria for histological classification, this histological distribution is different from that described by Ueda *et al.* (*27*) for 95 cases of ovarian cancer in the Osaka district, of which 68 (71.6%), 7 (7.4%), and 19 (20.0%) were for categories I, II, and IV,

TABLE IV.   Distribution of Ovarian Cancer by Histological Type and Exposure Dose

Histological type (WHO 1973)	Total		T65 dose in rad				
			0	1–99	100+	Unknown	NIC[a]
I. Common epithelial tumors	121	(94.5%)	50	35	12	1	23
A. Serous	61		26	17	7	1	10
B. Mucinous	27		12	7	2	0	6
C. Endometrioid	18		8	4	1	0	5
D. Clear cell	9		2	3	2	0	2
G. Undifferentiated carcinoma	2		0	2	0	0	0
H. Unclassified malignancy	4		2	2	0	0	0
II. Sex cord stromal tumors	4	(3.1%)	1	1	0	0	2
A. Granulosa cell	4		1	1	0	0	2
IV. Germ cell tumors	3	(2.3%)	0	0	0	0	3
F. Teratomas	3		0	0	0	0	3
Total	128	(100.0%)	51	36	12	1	28

[a] Not in city ATB.

respectively (one case belonged to a category other than I–IV). These distributions should also be compared to that reported by Yaker and Benirschke (*29*) in 74 cases in the San Diego district, which was 66 (89.2%), 2 (2.7%), and 6 (8.1%), respectively.

The histological distribution of the 79 combined nonexposed and 0 rad group cases is not significantly different from that of the 49 cases exposed to 1 rad or more, namely, 48 carcinomas of category I and one granulosa cell tumor of category II. Of the 48 carcinomas among the exposed cases, serous adenocarcinoma accounted for 52.1%, followed in order by mucinous adenocarcinoma and endometrioid carcinoma. Of the 12 cases among those that were exposed to 100 or more rad, 7 were serous adenocarcinoma, 2 mucinous adenocarcinoma, 1 endometrioid carcinoma, and 2 clear cell carcinoma. Of 7 in the 12 cases exposed to 200 or more rad, 4 were serous adenocarcinoma, 1 mucinous adenocarcinoma, and 2 clear cell carcinoma. In 3 out of the 12 cases exposed to 300 or more rad, 2 were serous adenocarcinoma and 1 was clear cell carcinoma. Thus there is no evidence of different histological type of carcinoma with varying magnitude of exposure dose.

Consider next the issue of benign tumors of the ovary. It is plausible that the clinical recognition of such benign tumors may be somewhat related to the frequency of receiving professional medical care. Were this conjecture true, one might expect the frequency of recognized benign tumors to be higher in exposed individuals, especially in those exposed to large doses, as these individuals would likely have received more frequent and intense medical care than nonexposed persons (due to the A-bomb Survivors Medical Treatment Law, *etc.*). In the autopsied series, there would be no such bias in the recognition of benign tumors of the ovary. A study was thus undertaken on benign ovarian tumors from 106 autopsied LSS cases of which 89 cases (84.0%) were reviewed microscopically. As shown in Table V, the proportion of autopsied cases with benign ovarian tumors increases with increasing exposure dose, both with the group of all 106 ascertained benign tumor cases ($p < 0.05$), and with the restricted subset of 89 microscopically reviewed cases, although statistical significance is not achieved in this latter group ($p > 0.10$).

Because tumors were bilateral in 9 cases, the total number of tumors amount to 98 in the 89 histologically reviewed cases. The histological distribution of these 98 tumors

TABLE V.   Age-adjusted Proportion of Subjects with Benign Ovarian Tumor Among
Autopsied Subjects (per 1,000) by Exposure Dose

Method of ascertainment	Total	T65 dose in rad						Test[b]
		0	1–49	50–99	100+	Unknown	NIC[a]	
Total	34.8	26.3	38.8	47.6	58.8	30.6	27.8	
	(106)	(22)	(48)	(8)	(11)	(1)	(16)	$p<0.05$
Histologically reviewed cases	29.2	21.5	34.1	35.1	42.2	29.9	24.3	
	(89)	(18)	(42)	(6)	(8)	(1)	(14)	$p>0.10$

The number in parentheses is the number of subjects with benign ovarian tumor.
[a] Not in city ATB.
[b] Statistical test for linear increase with dose (excluding unknown and NIC).

TABLE VI.   Distribution of Autopsied Benign Ovarian Tumors by
Histological Type and Exposure Dose

Histological type (WHO 1973)	Total		T65 dose in rad				
			0	1–99	100+	Unknown	NIC[a]
I. Common epithelial tumors	60	(61.2%)	12	37	2	1	8
A. Serous	49		9	33	2	0	5
B. Mucinous	5		3	0	0	1	1
C. Endometrioid	1		0	1	0	0	0
E. Brenner	5		0	3	0	0	2
II. Sex cord stromal tumors	17	(17.3%)	3	8	3	0	3
b. Fibroma	16		2	8	3	0	3
c. Sclerosing stromal	1		1	0	0	0	0
IV. Germ cell tumors	21	(21.4%)	5	9	3	0	4
2. Mature cystic teratoma	19		3	9	3	0	4
3. Struma ovarii	2		2	0	0	0	0
Total	98	(100.0%)	20	54	8	1	15

[a] Not in city ATB.

is shown in Table VI. Of the 35 tumors occurring in the combined nonexposed and 0 rad groups, the number (and percentage) in categories I, II, and IV are 20 (57.1%), 6 (17.1%), and 9 (25.7%), respectively. This histologic distribution is not significantly different from that of the 63 tumors in cases exposed to 1 or more rad, namely, 40 (63.5%), 11 (17.5%), and 12 (19.0%) in categories I, II, IV, respectively. Comparison can also be made with other reported histologic distributions: 177 (45.2%), 20 (5.1%), and 193 (49.2%) among 392 tumors (including two cases in other than categories I–IV) in the Osaka district (27); 54 (46.6%), 14 (12.1%), and 48 (41.4%) among 116 tumors in San Diego (29); 637 (62.5%), 75 (7.4%), and 297 (29.1%) among 1,019 tumors (including 10 cases in other than categories I–IV) in Montreal (2). Thus, the distribution in this study does not differ significantly from reports mentioned above, except those in Osaka.

Experiments in radiation tumorigenesis have shown that ovarian tumors of several histological types can be induced in mice of various strains. For example, single dose whole-body irradiation of $(C57L \times A/He)F_1$ mice with gamma rays or neutrons induced various ovarian tumors, including luteoma, granulosa cell tumor, and adenoma (28). Similarly, single dose whole-body X-ray irradiation induced luteomas and adenomas in the ovaries of ddY/F and C3H/Tw mice (12).

It has been suggested that ionizing radiation primarily induces atrophy of follicles in the mouse ovary (14), and the consequent imbalanced hormonal environment, due to excessive gonadotropic hormone secretion, plays a significant role in the tumorigenesis of the ovary (13). In this regard, Furth (8) stated that a series of changes, namely, atrophy of the ovary due to radiation exposure, the secondary excess of gonadotrophic hormones, and changes in the response of cells that comprise the injured ovary, facilitate the development of ovarian tumors.

According to the study by Tokunaga et al. (25), breast cancer incidence in exposed females of Hiroshima and Nagasaki shows a linear dose response, and the age specific incidence of breast cancer exceeds that of breast cancer in the general female population. However, both the trend of the cumulative incidence with time and the histological distribution of breast cancer closely resemble that of breast cancer in general. These findings are consistent with the hypothesis that postexposure endogenous hormones act as tumor promoters in the genesis of breast cancer in A-bomb female survivors (25).

The pathological and epidemiological analyses described herein of the 194 cases of ovarian cancer that had occurred during 1950–80 among LSS members strongly suggest that the incidence of ovarian cancer was enhanced by A-bomb exposure; moreover, the radiation-related excess of ovarian cancer appears to be highest in women less than 20 years of age when exposed, with these women having the longest latent period compared to the older age groups. The histological distribution of cancer types among exposed individuals appears not very different from that seen in the general population. As for benign ovarian neoplasms, the analysis of 106 autopsy subjects depicts a trend of increasing radiation-related tumor excess with increasing dose among the exposed cases, though the trend is not statistically significant when observation was limited to the histologically reviewed cases.

From experimental findings concerning the induction of ovarian tumors by ionizing radiation and from recent analysis of breast carcinogenesis in exposed females of Hiroshima and Nagasaki, one might deduce that radiation injury in association with secondary excess of gonadotrophic hormones is an important causative factor in the development of ovarian tumors in the Hiroshima and Nagasaki female survivors; the pathological and epidemiological findings detailed herein are consistent with this hypothesis. Further follow-up studies should therefore be made on females who were exposed to the A-bomb at the younger ages, particularly at ages less than 20 years when exposed.

REFERENCES

1. Anderson, M. R. and Jackson, S. H. Long term follow-up of patients with menorrhagia treated by irradiation. Br. J. Radiol., 44, 295–298 (1971).
2. Beck, R. P. and Latour, J.P.A. Review of 1019 benign ovarian neoplasms. Obstet. Gynecol., 16, 479–482 (1960).
3. Boice, J. D., Jr., Day, N. E., Andersen, A., Brinton, L. A., Brown, P., Choi, N. W., Clarke, E. A., Colemen, M. P., Curtis, R. E., Flannery, J. T., Hakama, M., Hakulinen, T., Howe, G. R., Jensen, O. M., Kleinerman, R. A., Magnin, D., Magnus, K., Makela, K., Malker, B., Miller, A. B., Nelson, N., Patterson, C. C., Pettersson, F., Pompe-Kirn, V., Primic-Zakelc, M., Prior, P., Ravnihar, P., Skeet, R. G., Skjerven, J. E., Smith, P. G., Sok, N., Spengler, R. F., Storm, H. H., Tomkins, G.W.O., Wall, C., and Weinstock, R. Cancer risk following radiotherapy of cervical cancer. In "Radiation Carcinogenesis: Epidemiology and Biological Significance: Progress in Cancer Research, Vol 26.," ed.

J. D. Boice, Jr. and J. F. Fraumeni, Jr., pp. 161–179 (1984). Raven Press, New York.

4. Conrad, R. A. Late radiation effects in Marshall Islanders exposed to fallout 28 years ago. *In* "Radiation Carcinogenesis: Epidemiology and Biological Significance: Progress in Cancer Research, Vol. 26," ed. J. D. Boice, Jr. and J. F. Fraumeni, Jr., pp. 57–71 (1984). Raven Press, New York.

5. Court Brown, W. M. and Doll, R. Mortality from cancer and other causes after radiotherapy for ankylosing spondylitis. *Br. Med. J.*, **2**, 1327–1332 (1965).

6. Crossen, R. J. and Crossen, H. S. Radiation therapy of uterine myoma: Critical analysis of results in 500 cases, showing indications and limitations. *J. Am. Med. Assoc.*, **133**, 593–599 (1947).

7. Dickson, R. J. The late results of radium treatment for benign uterine hemorrhage. *Br. J. Radiol.*, **42**, 582–594 (1969).

8. Furth, J. Radiation neoplasia and endocrine system. *In* "Radiation Biology and Cancer," pp. 7–25 (1959). University of Texas Press, Austin.

9. Hiroshima City Medical Association: Epidemiological observation of malignant neoplasms in the atomic bomb survivors in Hiroshima. 1. *Hiroshima Med. J.*, **14**, 347–356 (1961).

10. Preston, D. L., Kato, H., Kopecky, K. J., and Fujita, S. Life Span Study, Report 10. Part I. Cancer mortality among atomic bomb survivors, 1950–82. RERF Tech. Rep. 1-86 (1986).

11. Kinutani, K. Two cases of the ovarian neoplasm developed in exposed women. *Hiroshima Med. J.*, **11**, 892–895 (1958) (in Japanese).

12. Kimuro, M. Ovarian tumorigenesis after whole-body X-ray irradiation in ddY/F and CH3/Tw mice. *J. Radiol. Res.*, **17**, 99–105 (1976).

13. Li, M. H. and Gardner, W. U. Experimental studies on the pathogenesis and histogenesis of ovarian tumors in mice. *Cancer Res.*, **7**, 549–566 (1947).

14. Lorenz, E. Some biologic effects of long continued irradiation. *Am. J. Roentgenol.*, **63**, 176–185 (1950).

15. Milton, R. C. and Shohoji, T. Tentative 1965 radiation dose estimation for atomic bomb survivors, Hiroshima and Nagasaki. *ABCC TR*, 1–68 (1968).

16. Novak, E. R. and Woodruff, J. D. Postirradiation malignancies of the pelvic organs. *Am. J. Obstet. Gynecol.*, **77**, 667–675 (1959).

17. Palmer, J. P. and Spratt, D. W. Pelvic carcinoma following irradiation for benign gynecological diseases. *Am. J. Obstet. Gynecol.*, **72**, 497–505 (1956).

18. Rubin, P., Ryplansky, A. and Dutton, A. Incidence of pelvic malignancies following irradiation for benign gynecologic conditions. *Am. J. Roentgenol.*, **85**, 503–514 (1961).

19. Sawada, H. Evaluation of gynecological tumors in the atomic bomb survivors. ABCC Tech. Rep. 6-59 (1959).

20. Serov, S. F. and Scully, R. E. "Histological Typing of Ovarian Tumours" (1973). World Health Organization, Geneva.

21. Smith, P. G. Late effects of X-ray treatment of ankylosing spondylitis. *In* "Radiation Carcinogenesis: Epidemiology and Biological Significance: Progress in Cancer Research, Vol. 26," ed. J. D. Boice and J. F. Fraumeni, Jr., pp. 107–118 (1984). Raven Press, New York.

22. Smith, P. G. and Doll, R. Late effects of X-irradiation in patients treated for metropathia hemorrhagica. *Br. J. Radiol.*, **49**, 224–232 (1976).

23. Tabuchi, A. Gynecological and obstetrical surveys on the atomic bomb survivors. *Hiroshima Med. J.*, **12**, 958–964 (1959) (in Japanese).

24. Thomas, W. O., Jr., Harris, H. H. and Enden, J. A. Postirradiation malignant neoplasms of the uterine fundus. *Am. J. Obstet. Gynecol.*, **104**, 209–219 (1969).

25. Tokunaga, M., Land, C. E., Yamamoto, T., Asano, M., Tokuoka, S., Ezaki, H., Nishimori, I. and Fujikura, T. Breast cancer among atomic bomb survivors. *In* "Radiation

Carcinogenesis: Epidemiology and Biological Significance: Progress in Cancer Research, Vol. 26," ed. J. D. Boice, Jr. and J. F. Fraumeni, Jr., pp. 45–56 (1984). Raven Press, New York.

26. Tokuoka, S., Kawai, K., Shimizu, Y., Kato, H., Ohe, K., Inai, K., and Fujikura, T. Malignant and benign ovarian neoplasms among atomic bomb survivors, Hiroshima and Nagasaki, 1950–80. RERF Tech. Rep., in preparation.

27. Ueda, G., Yamasaki, M., Inoue, M., and Kurachi, K. A clinicopathologic study of ovarian tumors. *Acta Obstet. Gynaecol. Jpn.*, **32**, 37–45 (1980) (in Japanese with English Abstr.)

28. Upton, A. C., Kimball, A. W., Furth, L., Christenberry, K. W., and Benedict, W. H. Some delayed effects of atom-bomb radiations in mice. *Cancer Res.*, **20** (8) Part 2, 1–60 (1960).

29. Yaker, A. and Benirschke, K. A ten year study of ovarian tumors. *Virchows Arch. A Pathol. Anat. Histopathol.*, **366**, 275–286 (1975).